Dedication

This book is fondly dedicated to Bob and Judy Stewart of Winnipeg and Ernie and Janet Welburn of Churchill, Manitoba. Bob and Judy have hosted our expeditions since 1972, helping us organize and head into the bush. Ernie and Janet have collected us in Churchill after our wilderness sojourns. Both families have stored gear, canoes, and memories and have patiently waited for our return—year after year—season after season.

Thanks for all your help. It enabled dozens of youngsters (and oldsters) to make our trips into the Arctic possible.

Doc

Contents

Preface

The greatest risk the outdoor traveler faces is accidental hypothermia, whether brought about slowly as a result of improper clothing during a cold and frequently wet land—based experience, or from a sudden cooling due to immersion in cold water.

This book was written to provide guidance in the event of such occurrences. Since the last edition of this book in 1991, several new field warming techniques have been studied. Rewarming the core temperature by immersing the hands and legs in warm water, a technique used by the Danish Navy since the 1970s, has been studied and found to be a safe method of adding heat (see page 62). Forced air rewarming systems have been developed and a new method of rewarming using negative pressure on the extremities has been shown effective in treating mild hypothermia (see page 62).

While a greater range of hospital-based rewarming methods are also being explored, the most effective methods for handling the wilderness hypothermia patient are still far from clear.

This book makes the point that it seems reasonable to consider the field classification of hypothermia as consisting of two basic situations: Hypothermia of rapid onset and hypothermia of slow onset. Each of these conditions can be further classified as mild or profound (severe). The reason for these classifications is to aid diagnosis and thus treatment in the field. Management techniques are discussed in the sections dealing with field treatments. These sections will be further referenced in this book's Web site at www.adventure-media.com/hypothermia/.

Hypothermia

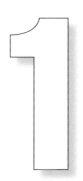

One of a human's most significant tasks is to maintain the internal, or core, temperature at a fairly even setting near 100°F (37°C). An environmental, or ambient, temperature lower than 77°F (25°C) results in a lowering of the core temperature of a naked human, unless either a mental or physiological response to counter that drop occurs.

Obviously a temperature gradient exists, nearly always, between the core and the outside temperature. We are able to tolerate temperatures, even in excess of our core temperature, by losing heat via evaporation. Heat is also lost through radiation—in fact 50 to 65 percent of our total heat output is normally lost via radiation alone. Convection is a method of heat loss only when there is a current of air or water washing past us, thereby removing the heat layer next to our body. Conduction loss is normally not much of a factor, unless we are pressing against a very cold object, or unless we find ourselves immersed in cold water.

 For a further discussion of this topic refer to Chapter 2, Physical Laws of Heat Transfer, on page 11.

Our method of responding to a cooler environment takes one of three forms. One is intellectual. We can change the environment by obtaining shelter, moving from a cold place to a warmer area, building a fire, putting on clothes, etc. An intellectual response also includes decreasing our surface area by rolling up into a ball (while sleeping in a cold sleeping bag, or assuming positions such as the HELP position used in cold water and discussed on page 71. It was an intellectual response to cold that allowed us to develop the technology of making clothing adequate to enable us to move from a tropical environment and to spew our population out over the entire surface of mother earth.

For a further discussion of this topic refer to Chapter 3, Protection from the Cold, on page 22.

Another response is to generate more heat internally. We constantly generate heat as we use the muscles necessary to breath and pump our blood. This energy requirement is called the basal metabolic rate (or BMR) and generally equals about 75 kcal (314 kJ) of energy per hour.

We must consume the amount of food that will allow us to produce this energy. In fact, we must consume slightly more food value than 75 kcal to allow for certain inefficiencies in converting the food to energy. This inefficiency is called the specific dynamic action of food (SDA) and it differs by the type of foodstuff and by the combinations of foodstuffs that we are consuming. The SDA ranges from 30 percent for pure protein to about 11 percent for a combination of fat, carbohydrate, and protein consumed together.

 For a further discussion of this topic refer to Chapter 4, Nutritional Requirements and Nonmuscular Heat Production, on page 36.

Fortunately we are capable of doing more work than just breathing, pumping blood, and eating. This additional work activity requires more energy and generates more heat. The ability to perform work, and the limit of our ability to generate various amounts of heat, is related to our level of physical conditioning. Other immediate influences on work/heat output are level of current nutrition, hydration, wellness, and rest. Shivering is a form of work in which very little is accomplished except the oscillation of muscles for the purpose of generating heat. Shivering is therefore limited by the amount of physical conditioning and the other factors that also determine how much actual work we are capable of performing.

 For a further discussion of this topic refer to Chapter 5, Muscular Heat Production, on page 45.

The third response to heat loss is a series of physiological responses. Top of the list in efficiency and importance is the ability of most arteries to narrow their diameter and constrict their blood flow. Called *vasoconstriction*, the blood flow can be selectively decreased to our skin surface and to our limbs. This prevents a significant amount of heat loss.

Vasoconstriction is controlled by both local (skin) receptors and by central controls in the brain. Placing a hand in ice water will cause vasoconstriction in that hand alone, while the return of cooler blood to the brain will produce a generalized vasoconstriction, thus effecting heat conservation.

 For a further discussion of this topic refer to Chapter 6, Physiological Responses to Prevent Heat Loss, on page 50.

The Development of Hypothermia

The battle to maintain our core at 98.6°F (37°C) is generally successful, except under two different scenarios that result in the illness we call hypothermia. The term *hypothermia* refers to two disease states that are quite different from each other. The pathology is different, the ideal treatment is different, and even the evaluation or prediction of severity of risk for these victims is different. These two disease states, which share the name hypothermia, both represent a lowered core temperature. The rate at which the core temperature is lowered causes the pathology or illness in victims to differ significantly. These two processes are called chronic hypothermia and acute hypothermia.

Chronic Hypothermia

Chronic hypothermia is the lowering of the core temperature below 95°F (35°C) over a period of six hours or longer. Chronic hypothermia can develop by simply not wearing adequate insulation to maintain thermal balance with the environment—in other words, by wearing clothes that are a little too light for the current temperature/wind conditions. At times light clothing is required, such as when working and thus producing excess heat that needs to be discharged to the environment. But when this extra work (skiing, cutting wood, etc.) is stopped, we become acutely aware of the need for a heavier jacket. If we are unable to obtain improved covering or shelter, we start a slow loss of heat to the environment, greater than the amount that we were producing. The gradual cooling that will result is minimized by the body causing vasoconstriction. If we are too exhausted to work, shivering is also not an option, for it, too, requires energy to function.

Generally a thermal balance results in which our decreased energy output/work production, clothing, and vasoconstriction allow the heat loss to slow to the point that it balances heat production. In case this does not prove to be possible, where the heat loss is greater than the amount of heat that we can produce and protect, a slow cooling

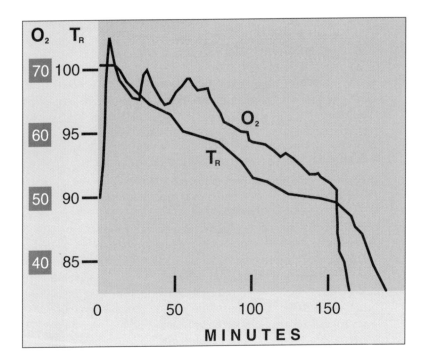

Figure 1-1

Sudden Loss of Core Temperature After Consumption of Energy Substrate.

The rectal temperature curve (32°) in this subject makes a sudden downward plunge at about the 90°F (32°C) point. As an indicator that this is due to the loss of energy substrate, note that oxygen consumption (O_2), which indicates the amount of energy substrate being used, and therefore available for use, has dropped simultaneously. (Oxygen consumption is shown in units of ml/kg/min and the temperature curve in Fahrenheit degrees.)

Source: Marlin Kreider, M.D., in *Appalachia*, Dec. 1980.

progresses. The cooling is usually slow, unless a catastrophic imbalance with the environment has occurred, such as a very profound temperature decrease, sudden soaking of all protective clothing, or immersion in cold water.

 For a further discussion of this topic refer to Chapter 7, Detection and Prevention of Chronic Hypothermia, on page 54.

If a gradual heat loss extends over hours, the net effect of massive vasoconstriction and subsequent fluid shifting into the core is a profound dehydration (even with adequate fluid intake) and a compacting and alteration of the blood to allow the tremendous decrease in blood volume that occurs. We can predict when this compacting of blood volume has become significant by the core temperature. As mentioned, a person is considered "hypothermic" when his core temperature drops to 95°F (35°C). At this core temperature level, and for several degrees below this, while the person is hypothermic, the blood fluid volume and its alterations are not profound. With continued cold exposure, eventually there will be a sudden decrease in the core temperature that basically is the result of the total exhaustion of the high energy subtrates required to maintain even this poor level of thermal balance. A core temperature of 90°F (32°C) marks the spot at which we consider the victim as being in profound, chronic hypothermia.

As seen in Figure 1-1, the core temperature drop is not linear. Rather it is flat initially as the protective mechanism of vasoconstriction and the resulting slowly decreasing thermal mass is at first maintained. It is only lost when exhaustion (loss of energy producing substrates) finally occurs.

The rescue of a chronic hypothermic individual requires the prevention of further heat loss regardless of the core temperature. Above a core temperature of 90°F (32°C), virtually any method of handling the victim is fine. Heat may be added rapidly or slowly; he may be allowed to engage in any activity that he wishes—the only problem is that this person is at or near exhaustion and should be provided with shelter, food, hydration, and rest.

Below a 90°F (32°C) core temperature, however, we must be very careful how we handle the victim. He is alive but has a potentially lethal disease that requires careful management in the field. Rapid heat replacement can be lethal as the lack of adequate blood fluid volume results in a "rewarming shock." The phenomena of "afterdrop" is probably not as important in a chronic hypothermic as the development of rewarming shock and metabolic imbalances. This person requres gentle handling, the slow addition of heat, hydration (if he can safely swallow), prevention of further heat loss, and litter evacuation—aided by the addition of carefully protected heat packs, warmed canteens or other warmed objects and, ideally, the use of heated aerosol mist as described in Chapter 8. In a pinch, when evacuation is not feasible, the rescuers may have to resort to huddling with the victim in a sleeping bag for warmth.

For a further discussion of this topic refer to Chapter 8, Field Treatment of Chronic Hypothermia, on page 58.

Acute Hypothermia

Depending upon the clothing worn, falling into cold water causes such a massive heat loss that the protective mechanisms described above are insufficient to prevent any significant amount of heat loss. The result is called *acute hypothermia*, which is generally described as hypothermia occurring in two hours or less. The heat loss noted in these people is linear—reflecting the almost total lack of any influence of the vasoconstriction that is taking place. The body is simply overwhelmed with the heat drain, and a cooling takes place at a rate that is predictable based upon the thermal conductance of human tissue, body size (ratio of mass to surface area), activity during immersion, the water temperature, and the protective clothing (or lack thereof) being worn.

Rapid cooling does not allow the body to compact the circulatory volume into the core. The profound heat loss rapidly cools the victim into unconsciousness and death before this can take place. Taking the most severe scenario, a person in a light outfit of clothes, or virtually none at all, falling into ice water, will cool to a lethal level within one hour and fifteen minutes. Death in very cold water can be instant if the victim has a gasp reflex while under the water surface or if the victim develops a lethal heart irregularity (ventricular fibrillation) due to the shock of the cold water. This sudden death, or sudden disappearance syndrome in cold water, is the exception rather than the rule.

The likelihood that a naked person can last in ice water for one and a quarter hours before dying is probably a longer time than many people would have guessed. Cooling occurs most rapidly when the victim is exposed to cold, moving water, such as during entrapment in a river, while attempting to swim or tread water, or when being subjected to breaking waves in an agitated sea. Muscle tissue cooling can progress so fast, that before the victim develops core hypothermia, there may be a loss of coordination and the ability to use arms or legs to assist in a rescue, or even to remain floating upright.

Cold water immersion victims are in real trouble before they have reached the predicted death point during their immersion. The amount of total thermal mass lost during the immersion is quite immense, as somewhat indicated by that straight line on the heat loss

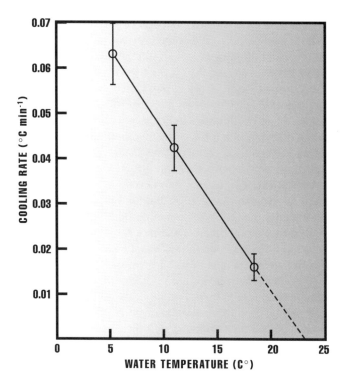

Figure 1-2

Linear Heat Loss of Core Temperature Resulting from Immersion.

Water temperature and the mean rectal temperature cooling rate in lightly clothed, nonexercising males and females during immersion in seawater are related.

Source: Hayward, "The Physiology of Immersion Hypothermia."
In Pozos and Wittmers, eds., *The Nature and Treatment of Hypothermia,*

graph. As a rule, a person who has been immersed longer than one-half of the time expected to reach his or her lethal end point is suffering from severe, or profound, acute hypothermia. See Figure 1-2.

 For a further discussion of this topic refer to Chapter 9, Detection and Prevention of Acute Hypothermia, on page 68.

The ideal treatment for this victim is rapid heat replacement, ideally in a hot water bath of 110°F (43°C), which will minimize the core afterdrop that will certainly continue after rescue from the immersion.

The afterdrop in an immersion victim can be profound. The amount of afterdrop in degrees can be predicted by the rate of cooling that was taking place at the time of rescue, but this can be blunted by the addition of massive amounts of heat, such as through the warm water immersion just mentioned. While warm water immersion would be life-threatening in the profound (core below 90°F or 32°C) chronic hypothermic, it can be lifesaving to the profound acute hypothermic. By definition it means that this person has been in cold water less than two hours. Persons immersed in cold water longer than two hours must be treated as chronic hypothermics and rapid heat replacement avoided. By the time that two hours has elapsed, victims have started developing dehydration and the physiological changes described under chronic hypothermia treatment in Chapter 8.

The immersion hypothermic is not suffering from a change in blood volume, or blood components, as is the case with the chronic hypothermic. However, the immersion hypothermic is suffering from a much more prodigious heat loss if a core temperature comparison is being made. The chronic hypothermic with a 90°F (32°C) core temperature is suffering from an approximate 500 kcal (2,000 kJ) heat deficit; while an acute hypothermic with the same core temperature reading could have a 1,200 kcal (5,000 kJ) heat deficit.

When rescuing the acute (generally immersion) hypothermic victim, the water temperature, length of time of exposure, activity of the victim, body size (ratio of surface area to mass), and percentage of body fat are the most important factors in evaluating the degree of hypothermia present, not simply the symptoms or even the core temperature of the victim. The estimate of whether a person is a profound, acute hypothermic can be simplified to looking at the length of time of immersion and the water temperature. Unless they are insulated with at least a wet suit, if the water temperature is 55°F (13°C) or colder and they have been in the water twenty minutes or longer, these victims are probably profound, acute hypothermics.

Persons considered as profound, acute hypothermics must not be allowed to run around. They are frequently capable of this, but it causes a massive movement of blood into the cold muscle mass in the extremities and back to the core. This results in a circulatory component of core afterdrop that adds to the impending conduction afterdrop that the cold surface tissues are about to cause anyway. However, they may not be simply wrapped in a sleeping bag without adding adequate heat, as their core temperature can continue cooling to a lethal level from conduction cooling due to the massive heat deficit from which they are suffering.

The significant concerns on the part of many rescuers and

researchers regarding the potential benefits versus risks of rapid rewarming by the hot water immersion treatment in profound, acute hypothermic victims are discussed in Chapter 10.

The importance of aggressively treating profound, acute hypothermic people, who appear so normal that they are able to walk, carry on conversations, and in all respects act as if they are not injured, has been stressed repeatedly. In 1980 sixteen Danish fishermen were forced to jump into the North Sea when their fishing boat floundered. They were in the water for about one and one-half hours before another boat was able to reach them. It lowered a cargo net to them. These men were still capable of climbing aboard via the net. They crossed the deck on their own and went below to the galley where they were supposed to have hot drinks and warm up. Instead, each one of these men died from hypothermia.

Constructing a huge fire is a good way to add an immense amount of heat in the field, especially when a tub of warm water is not convenient. At times it also may be impossible to start a large fire. The treatment is then simply to prevent further heat loss and to add heat in the best manner possible. This might amount to adding heat packs, warmed and wrapped canteens or rocks, etc., or to cuddle two rescuers with the victim in a sleeping bag—the very method that might have to be used as an ideal treatment for the profound, chronic hypothermic. It is not the ideal treatment for the profoundly acute hypothermic, as it is best to add heat to this victim as rapidly as possible.

Persons falling into cold water, with marginally protective gear on, may cool so slowly as to actually become chronic hypothermics. If rescued six hours into their ordeal, they are classic chronic hypothermics for they have had time to physiologically respond to the heat loss in a controlled, slow manner. In fact, a rescue after two hours means that the physiological changes seen in the chronic hypothermic are progressing and the use of hot water immersion as a treatment becomes more and more risky. The status of hypothermia onset between two and six hours has been called *sub-acute hypothermia*. It is best to arrange treatment of these people based upon the end of the spectrum that they seem the closest to matching.

All persons considered to have suffered profound hypothermia, be it acute or chronic, should be seen by a physician. These are very dangerous conditions that require adequate field management by you and then evacuation to a medical facility.

Low reading thermometers are available, but their use is not practical under most field conditions. The field decisions on how to treat these victims, and the urgency of the care needed, must frequently be made based primarily upon the length of exposure of the immersion victim and the symptoms of the chronic victim.

 For a further discussion of this topic refer to Chapter 10, Field Treatment of Acute Hypothermia and Submersion, on page 73.

Other Cold Injuries

Persons who develop hypothermia do not always develop frostbite, but they are at an increased risk of doing so. Similarly, persons with frostbite are not always hypothermic. These cold weather injuries each have their own risk factors, some of which overlap. The most notable increased risks common to these conditions are dehydration, shock or injury, being wet, decreased heat output (generally from exhaustion), and constricting garments.

The cold weather injuries of frostbite, immersion foot, chilblains, and frozen lung are discussed in Chapter 11.

The prevention of the cold weather injuries requires knowledge of how to avoid them, and frequently, proper pretrip planning to adequately prepare for the activity that you are about to undertake.

 For a further discussion of this topic refer to Chapter 11, Frostbite and Other Cold-Related Injuries, on page 78.

Physical Laws of Heat Transfer

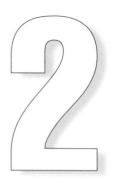

I n our daily lives and during our wilderness excursions, we must learn to take advantage of the physical laws relating to heat transfer. Even in a cold environment, preventing heat buildup is frequently necessary, primarily to prevent sweating and subsequent dampening of clothing, which causes loss of insulation efficiency.

The physical methods of heat transfer include radiation, conduction, evaporation, and convection. Variations of these basic physical events are loss through the physiology of respiration and the bellows effect of clothing and sleeping bags.

Radiation

Heat is discharged directly from the body by the emission of infrared energy. Actually, radiation heats a surrounding microenvironment that convection can then strip away from the body. Radiation can also add heat to the body directly from the sun, or through reflection, even from snow fields, and from other sources of radiant energy. Fires can provide radiant warmth, as well as convection heat from hot air.

Areas of potential loss will be those areas that are: (1) exposed to the environment, (2) have large blood supplies, and (3) are unable to restrict or minimize local blood supply significantly to prevent radiant heat loss. The uncovered head can lose up to one-half of the body's total heat production at 39°F (4°C).

Protection from radiation loss can be best accomplished by any occlusive covering. Plastic sheeting with a fine film of aluminum was developed in the mid-1960s to reflect infrared radiation loss. It is very likely that these "space blankets" provide very little radiation loss protection (see page 34).

Conduction

Conduction is the direct transfer of heat from one object to another. Conductive heat loss from a human is most often the direct transfer of heat from the body to a cold surface, such as snow, cold ground, or water. Reduction of conductive heat loss is through insulation.

Insulation is generally a form of trapped air space. A large air space will allow heat drain by convection, so for the air space to be an effective insulator, it must be divided into multiple, small cells. For example, sleeping on an air mattress on the cold ground provides only slight insulation, while the same thickness of a foam pad can provide considerable protection. The degree of heat loss due to conduction will depend upon the surface area of the individual exposed to the "cold surface," the quality of insulation between the two, and the temperature of both the individual's skin surface and the cold surface.

Table 2-1
....
Thermal Conductivity of Various Substances

Substance	Conductivity*	Temp. Measured (°C)
Air	.006	0°
Down	.01	20°
Polyester (Hollow)	.016	
Polyester (Solid)	.019	
Cotton	.033	
Snow (Old)	.115	0°
Cork	.128	30°
Sawdust	.14	30°
Wool Felt	.149	40°
Cardboard	.5	20°
Wood	.8	20°
Dry Sand	.93	20°
Water	1.4	12°
Brick	1.5	20°
Concrete	2.2	20°
Ice	5.7	0°

*Conductivity is the quantity of heat in gram calories transmitted per second through a plate of material 1 cm thick and 1 square cm in area when the temperature difference between the sides of the plate is 1°C.

The most extreme conduction loss can potentially occur when submerged in cold water. An immersed individual in still water will lose heat by conduction at a rate twenty times faster than a dry individual in still air at the same temperature. This loss is so profound that it can cause the rapid development of hypothermia in a victim immersed in water colder than 68°F (20°C), a condition termed *acute hypothermia.* This differs from the "chronic hypothermia" that outdoor travelers can develop from other than immersion situations. By definition, acute hypothermia develops in less than two hours. Acute hypothermia can generally be regarded as synonymous with "immersion hypothermia." The term *sub-acute hypothermia* has been applied to cases that develop between two to six hours. The physiological status of the sub-acute hypothermic victim will more closely correspond to either the acute or the chronic process depending upon which end of the time spectrum one finds the victim.

Many insulating materials lose their protective properties when wet. Wool is one of the best insulating materials available, yet when it absorbs one-third of its weight it loses much of its insulation capability. Cotton is a very poor insulator even when merely damp. Its use in the outdoors, even in denim jeans, should be avoided. The use of cotton clothing can and does lead to survival tragedies due to its poor insulating ability. See Table 2-1, a list of different substances and their ability to prevent heat loss through conductivity.

Conduction can be an insidious method of heat loss. Many people have heard that snow is a good insulator. But this insulation is at or below 32°F (0°C). If the local temperature has been –20° for several days, then the snow is –20° in that area. Plunging along with inadequate foot insulation in snow of that temperature can lead to disaster.

Increasing the surface of contact with the ground, such as by sitting or lying down, means more heat will be lost than if a small area of contact, such as the foot, is involved. Many types of clothing have insulation that can be crushed when lying on it. If this were to happen, the trapped air space is decreased and the insulating ability of the material is compromised. When resting on the ground, treat that cold ground as an enemy and expect that your clothing will frequently be inadequate protection when crushed against it. In an emergency, full use of "relatively" better insulation than surface rocks, packed earth, or snow must be attempted by using insulated pads, sleeping bags, extra clothing, packs, branches, leaves and grass, or even loose dirt beneath the victim. Bottom line, try to provide as much protection as possible against a continuous heat loss by conduction from the victim to the ground.

Hypothermia   13

Evaporation

When water changes from a liquid to a gas it must absorb heat called the "latent heat of vaporization" or "latent heat of evaporation" to accomplish this change in its physical state. There is no change in the temperature of the substance, but there is an energy requirement to make the change from a liquid to a gaseous state. This results in the consumption, or loss, of heat. While this is a valuable method of lowering body core temperature during times of high heat stress, it can become a liability during cold weather. The latent heat of vaporization is 0.54 kcal (2.26 kJ) per gram of water, or 245 kcal per pound (2,250 kJ/kg). This represents a considerable loss of heat and significant energy consumption if that heat must be replaced. As chopping firewood for an hour produces approximately 290 kcal (1,200 kJ) of heat, it can be readily seen that several pounds of water in winter clothing can result in a terrible loss of heat and energy.

While sweating is a primary means for the body to purposely reduce heat loss through the principle of latent heat of vaporization, this same principle may cost the body precious heat when wet clothes are drying on the victim, or moisture is drying from exposed skin surfaces. The production of sweat or the accidental wetting of clothing from the environment can thus reduce the effectiveness of insulation in two ways. One way is through heat consumed by water during the evaporation process. The other way is through increased conduction through wet, less effective insulation. Rescue methods should attempt to prevent unnecessary loss of heat due to the evaporation process. A method strongly advocated is to place the wet victim in a plastic (or otherwise water impermeable) barrier to prevent evaporation. Rescuers should take care to also provide additional dry insulation, if possible, to help prevent continued heat loss through conduction because wet insulation, even the most sophisticated modern fabrics, still loses considerable thermal resistance efficiency.

Latent heat of vaporization is entirely separate from the heat required to thaw frozen water. This is called the "latent heat of crystallization," but it plays virtually no significant role, even in the rescue of a victim with frozen clothing. In fact, frozen sleeping bags, or a shell of frozen clothing on a recent immersion victim in subfreezing weather, can aid the survival process by producing a windproof barrier. The latent heat of crystallization is potentially significant when dealing with the eating of snow. This subject is discussed further on page 44.

Convection

Both water and air are generally not still and thus another mechanism of heat loss can occur—loss by convection. The body is constantly warming a thin layer of water or air next to it, thus forming a micro-environment with a higher temperature that surrounds it and protects it from the lower ambient temperature of the environment. The slightest disturbance of this thin layer of warmth strips it away by convection. Thus, this warm layer of air or water is removed easily by wind, current, or by body movement and this heat is lost. This micro-layer must then be reheated. A continuous stripping action of the micro-environment will cause a continuous loss of heat from the body.

The importance of wind or water movement is hard to emphasize adequately. At very cold ambient temperatures, considerable heat loss will result from warming of the micro-environment. Movement of an air mass greatly accelerates this loss and, hence, the importance of the windchill table demonstrating a relative temperature level. This type of table puts the danger of the cold/wind combination into terms that are commonly understood, namely degrees above or below zero Fahrenheit.

This expression of *windchill factor* has been a great aid in warning people of the dangers of convection coupled with cold ambient temperature. It is based upon work performed by C. F. Passel and P. A. Siple in the Antarctic during the winter of 1941. In their experiment the time to freeze cylinders of water was measured under different cold weather conditions. They developed a formula that expressed heat loss as a function of wind speed and air temperature. As mentioned above, in the United States this expression is given in degrees above or below zero Fahrenheit. Table 2-2 shows a windchill factor chart using these terms and illustrates the danger to exposed flesh at various windchill temperatures.

U.S. Windchill charts have been developed from mathematical application of the National Weather Service formula (Technical Procedures Bulletin No. 165, June 15, 1976), commonly called the *Siple equation*. This equation has an error in that wind speeds at very low levels demonstrate an exaggerated heat loss, while wind speeds above 45 mph (72 km/hr) seem to cause little additional effect. This is not true, but many windchill charts which you will see will indicate "Wind speeds above 40 mph have little additional effect." With regard to both comfort and amount of heat loss, winds above this speed DO cause increasing heat loss at a particular temperature, but for practical purposes this well-established method of depicting the relative effect of wind speed on temperature has proven to be a valuable aid.

The windchill factor used in the United States should be more

TEMPERATURE FAHRENHEIT

Wind Speed MPH	50	40	35	30	25	20	15	10	5	0	-5	-10	-15	-20	-25	-30	-35	-40	-45	-50	-55	-60
CALM	50	40	35	30	25	20	15	10	5	0	-5	-10	-15	-20	-25	-30	-35	-40	-45	-50	-55	-60
5	48	37	33	27	21	16	12	6	1	-5	-11	-15	-20	-26	-31	-36	-41	-47	-52	-57	-65	-70
10	40	28	22	16	9	4	-2	-9	-15	-24	-27	-33	-38	-46	-52	-58	-64	-70	-75	-83	-90	-95
15	36	22	16	11	4	-2	-11	-18	-25	-32	-40	-45	-51	-58	-65	-72	-77	-85	-90	-99	-105	-110
20	32	18	12	4	-3	-10	-17	-24	-31	-39	-46	-53	-60	-67	-75	-82	-88	-96	-102	-110	-115	-120
25	30	16	9	1	-7	-15	-22	-29	-37	-44	-52	-59	-65	-75	-83	-88	-96	-104	-111	-118	-125	-135
30	28	13	6	-2	-11	-18	-26	-33	-41	-48	-56	-63	-70	-79	-87	-94	-101	-109	-115	-125	-130	-140
35	27	11	5	-4	-13	-20	-27	-35	-43	-51	-60	-67	-72	-82	-90	-98	-105	-113	-120	-129	-135	-146
40	26	10	1	-6	-15	-21	-29	-37	-45	-53	-62	-69	-76	-85	-94	-100	-107	-115	-125	-132	-140	-150

Exposed flesh can freeze in 60 seconds

Exposed flesh can freeze in 30 seconds

Table 2-2

Windchill Equivalent Temperature – Fahrenheit

Note 1. The above chart has been based upon the Siple Equation and reflects windchill equivalent temperatures in Fahrenheit.

Note 2. At low wind speeds, relative humidity and radiant heat are more important than wind speed in determining equivalent temperature comfort.

Note 3. Most charts indicate that at wind speeds over 40 mph there is little additional wind chill effect. This reflects an error in the basic equation at these higher wind speeds and is not correct. Heat loss is magnified by these higher wind speeds, but the chart is an accurate indicator of equivalent temperature at speeds lower than 40 mph.

correctly termed an "equivalent chill temperature" or ECT. The windchill factor is actually a reflection of the rate of cooling due to convection heat loss. It is not an actual temperature. Some people assume incorrectly that objects can cool down to the windchill equivalent temperature if left outside. This is not possible as objects will NOT cool to a lower temperature than the surrounding ambient (local air) temperature.

In Canada, where the use of metric has supplanted the miles per hour for wind speed and the Celsius degree has replaced the Fahrenheit degree, a different expression of windchill is used. The expression "watts per square meter per hour" is an accurate expression of the actual energy loss due to the movement of air and the ambient temperature. The term seems foreign to the American ear, as I am sure it did to the Canadian ear when they first converted to the metric system. But like all systems, with use one readily identifies the perceived degree of coldness with the windchill factor, whether it is expressed in "windchill equivalent degrees Fahrenheit" or "watts per square meter per hour."

The advantage to the Canadian system is that the value actually expresses the amount of heat loss. This heat loss is in watts, a term that describes energy. The normal expression of metabolic energy is "kilocalorie." We generally call kilocalories "calories." Throughout this book I have used the more correct expression *kilocalories* and abbreviate it "kcal." Watts can be converted to kcal by multiplying watts by .862. By using the Canadian windchill chart, one can demonstrate the actual energy loss that can be converted to the number of kcal required to supply the amount of heat involved.

When using the Canadian windchill chart several factors should be remembered. First, the table has been derived from the Siple equation, again showing some of the inaccuracies of very low wind speeds and of wind speeds above 45 mph (72 km/hr). Second, the energy loss is computed per square meter of skin exposed. Of course, a square meter of skin would not be exposed during cold temperatures. The average adult male has 1.8 square meters of skin on his entire body. Only a small area of bare skin, namely parts of the head and occasionally the hands, would be exposed under very cold conditions.

At times nomograms are used in computing windchill values. Figure 2-1 is a well-known Canadian nomogram for calculating windchill values in watts per square meter per hour. A major value in computing the windchill factor is the determination of the degree of comfort and danger during exposure to the combined effects of temperature and wind speed. A general idea of the windchill factor significance can be found by the table accompanying the nomogram.

Hypothermia

The immense amount of heat loss due to immersion in cold water is discussed in sections on conduction and cold water immersion. Movement of water, or of the individual through water, also causes a convection heat loss. This has caused the development of special techniques for floating in cold water to minimize heat loss and increase survival chances (see section on Cold Water Submersion, page 76).

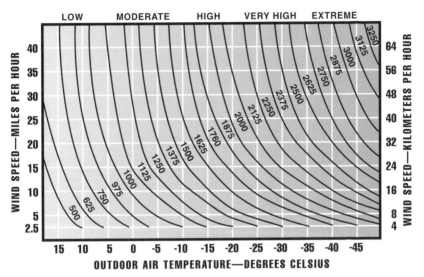

Factor	Comments
700	Conditions considered comfortable when dressed for skiing.
1200	Conditions no longer pleasant for outdoor activities on overcast days.
1400	Conditions no longer pleasant for outdoor activities on sunny days.
1600	Freezing of exposed skin begins for most people depending on the degree of activity and the amount of sunshine.
2300	Conditions for outdoor travel such as walking become dangerous. Exposed areas of the face freeze in less than one minute for the average person.
2700	Exposed flesh will freeze within half a minute for the average person.

For windchill follow the temperature across and the wind speed up until the two lines intersect. Below 8 k/hr it is difficult to determine windchill because factors such as relative humidity become important.

Figure 2-1

Windchill Cooling Rates (Watts per Square Meter).

The actual windchill cooling rates in watts per square meter per hour can be computed from the above graph. This figure can be converted into kcal of energy loss or windchill comfort as indicated in the text. *(Reproduced courtesy of Canada, Department of the Environment, Atmospheric Environmental Service.)*

Physiological Mechanisms Allowing Heat Loss

In addition to the physical laws that govern heat exchange, there are certain physiological actions that contribute directly to heat loss.

Respiration Heat Loss

Maintenance of life requires respiration primarily for oxygen exchange. Activity of any kind increases the rate or depth of respiration. Cold air must be warmed and humidity increased by the upper airways of the nose, the nasal and oral pharynx, to 100 percent humidity and virtually core temperature to prevent drying and cold vasospasm of bronchial and lung tissue. Figure 2-2 shows the calculation of heat loss due to respiration.

Air Temperature	Convective Heat Loss For Average Man kcal/hour	kJ/hour	
68°F (20°C)	5.8	24	Add 24.3 kcal/hour (102 kJ/hour) Evaporative heat loss
32°F (0°C)	12.5	52	
-4°F (-20°C)	19.3	80	
-40°F (-40°C)	26.	190	

HEAT LOSS DURING RESPIRATION

Figure 2-2

Heat Loss During Respiration.
Convective heat loss from warming air varies directly with the outside air temperature. The evaporative heat loss of respiration is a steady loss of 24.3 kcal/hour (102 kJ/hour), which is independent of temperature and which must be added to the figures.

The evaporative heat loss from providing humidity to expired air varies with the relative humidity of the outside air and the rate of respiration. Assuming a respiratory rate of 1.4 kilograms of air per hour, at temperatures below freezing, the rather dry relative humidity remains constant for this calculation and would result in a fairly steady heat loss of 24.3 kcal (102 kJ/hr). This amount of energy loss should be added to the above table to determine the total heat loss due to respiration.

This air has been heated and humidity increased at a cost and when expelled it represents a source of lost body heat. This mechanism is so important in some mammals that it represents their primary method of cooling the body during heat stress (for example, the panting dog).

Bellows Effect

Movement of an individual will increase convection loss. But movement also produces the *bellows effect*. This phenomenon is familiar to all winter campers. The slightest movement in a sleeping bag briefly blows hot air out and sucks cold air in. This movement also allows heat loss from parkas. To compensate for this, manufacturers tend to place elastic wrist cuffs in garments. In cold weather camping any restriction of peripheral blood flow increases the change of frost bite. To avoid this problem the Inuit (Eskimo) place a fur rim around the edge of parka sleeves and also attach a fur inner cuff to heavy mittens. They can thus place their hands easily into mittens, which are attached to a cord that hangs out their sleeves, the fur plugging any air movement with no restriction of blood flow.

The parka bellows effect around the neck is generally decreased in bulky garments due to their tight fit on the upper torso and at the shoulders.

A fur trimmed hood on a parka can form a breathing tunnel, or snorkel, for cold weather use that will reduce the bellows effect, prevent much direct wind conduction loss, decrease respiration heat losses, and block radiation loss from the head. Any parka designed for serious winter use must have a generous hood, preferably with a frost resistant trim.

Major Artery Heat Loss

If a major blood vessel were to come close to the skin, it would be in danger of allowing unnecessary heat loss during bitter cold conditions. The Inuit apparently knew of the importance of the femoral artery, which travels from deep in the abdomen to relatively near the surface of the front aspect of the leg beneath the inguinal ligaments. It is for this reason that they developed short outer pants that provide additional thermal protection to this vital artery. These pants could easily be removed, since they were worn over their trousers and were large enough to easily slip over footwear. Conversely, the groin is an excellent area to apply heat during field rewarming of a hypothermic victim.

Other areas of major artery heat loss are the axilla (armpit), neck, and in both flanks due to the kidney locations being near the surface there. These are all areas that should be protected from heat loss and that also make good locations to add heat when treating the hypothermic victim.

Urinary Heat Loss

Urinating seems an awful waste of body heat, but a quick calculation demonstrates that this loss is not significant. The average urinary output per day is approximately 1,500 ml (1.6 quarts). It takes 55½ kcal (233 kJ) to heat that quantity of water from freezing to body core temperature. Water drunk warmer could cause less of a heat loss, but the unusual aspect of cold weather travel is the tremendous desire for a very cold drink of water. Due to this rather low energy requirement, drinking cold water is not harmful during winter travel in the healthy individual.

Shiver Heat Loss

As mentioned elsewhere, shivering is a primary method of increasing heat production in the body. However, this activity causes increased blood flow to muscle mass, vasodilation, and an increase in potential bellows effect. Shivering results in a 25 percent increase in body heat loss. As shivering can increase heat production from 200 to 500 percent, it is still a valuable heat-generating technique. But minimizing potential losses during the shivering process can make it more valuable.

Cold-Induced Vasolidation Heat Loss

A method of preventing frostbite is a periodic expansion (vasodilation) of the arteries. This carries the fancy term *cold-induced vasodilation*, but it is frequently called the "hunting response." At a tissue temperature of 59°F (15°C), vasoconstriction will be maximal. If the tissue cools further to 50°F (10°C), intermittent periods of vasodilation occur to apparently provide some protection to tissues from frostbite and anoxia (or low oxygen supply). This, however, does allow a slight heat loss. The body has sacrificed a portion of the heat preservation aspect of vasoconstriction to preserve the life of the tissues involved. Periodic vasodilation is an insignificant source of heat loss.

Protection from the Cold

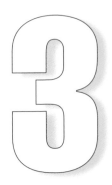

The use of shelters and clothing has made it possible for us to survive in nontropical environments. Earliest man had to get by with simply seeking refuge under trees, rocks, or other makeshift windbreaks. The ability to produce an artificial covering for our bodies was a significant achievement, ranking right behind learning you could smack things with "tools" like a chunk of rock and carry water away from its source in a gourd or other container. With garments as simple as raw skins or protective mats made of plants, the true age of exploration began. It has only been since the 1940s that we added synthetic, "man-made" fibers to treated animal skins and natural fibers in clothing construction.

Clothing allows you to carry your house on your back. Inuit hunters are able to stand over seal breathing holes on a windswept ice shelf for over a day in bitter cold Arctic conditions because they know what skin clothing to use. For millennia hunters have had to spend days away from their camps, using only their clothing and makeshift shelters for protection. While physiological responses to temperature provide protection above 77°F (25°C), it is our intellectual response to cold that allows us to survive at colder temperatures. This response consists of producing and seeking shelter or appropriate clothing.

Clothing Insulation—the "Clo"

The insulation value of a garment is measured in a unit called a *clo*. The value of 1 clo is approximately the insulation provided by a normal business suit. The actual thermal resistance of the value of a clo can be described mathematically. Thermal resistance represents the property of a material to prevent the flow of heat from a warm body to a cold environment.

All of us have received outdoor equipment catalogs and have noted that sleeping bags and garments are frequently rated with a comfort range. The catalog may claim that a particular bag is good to 20°F (-6°C), 0°F (-17.7°C), or so forth. But when using this item in the field, we may find that we have a difference of opinion! This is not the manufacturer's fault, it simply reflects an inherent difference in people. Some people simply sleep warmer than others. Factors involved are the basal metabolic rate, amount of subcutaneous fat for insulation, psychological attitude, body surface area, and many minor determinants.

Wouldn't it be ideal to have a foolproof rating system? One that manufacturers, advertisers, and consumers could all agree upon? Any such method should be based on the actual insulation, or the thermal resistance unit of any garment or equipment. The *clo* provides this ability. The building construction trade measures insulation using the term *R Factor*. These two terms are convertible; to change an R Factor value to a clo, multiply the R factor by 1.136. To go the other direction, multiply the clo by .88. Even a standardized system such as the clo does not directly indicate a comfort range; rather, it precisely indicates the amount of resistance to nonevaporative heat loss per unit of surface area to provide a comfortable skin temperature of 89.6°F (32°C). With experience consumers would soon realize precisely what clo rating they personally require to be comfortable under various temperature conditions while engaged in different activities.

The total insulation of garments is cumulative. If the clo value of various articles is known, add these values together to compute the total insulation provided by the ensemble. Figure 3-1 indicates the control of nonevaporative heat loss at different levels of activity and ambient temperatures.

From Figure 3-1 it can be seen that a man at rest, generating 108 kcal (450 kJ) per hour of metabolic heat at this activity level, will require about 1 clo unit of insulation to be in thermal balance at 68°F (20°C). If the temperature were to drop to 32°F (0°C), he would require approximately 2.3 clo, and with a further temperature drop to -4°F (-20°C), his requirement would be 4.3 clo. However, an active skier generating 290 kcal (1,200 kJ) of heat production due to his activity level would only need clothing that provided an effective clo of 2 even at a much lower temperature of -25°F (-31°C).

Clothing Construction, Materials, and Techniques

The clo value of a garment is dependent upon the material from which it is constructed and its design. Easily compressed insulation,

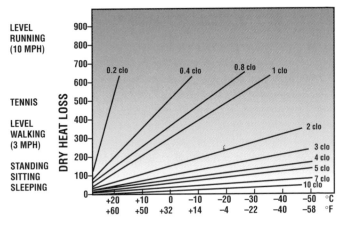

Figure 3-1
....

Heat Loss versus Clo Factor at a Comfortable Skin Temperature

The use of different insulation amounts, expressed in clo factors, that would allow nonevaporative heat loss in kcal/hour for a standard sized man at different temperature ranges and activity levels to keep his skin a constant warm temperature (89.6°F or 32°C).

Source: **3M Corporation.**

such as down, will lose its effectiveness at pressure points, such as the shoulders if a jacket hangs heavily upon the wearer. To prevent the problem of compression of insulation under sleeping bags against the cold ground, one needs less compressible insulation on the underside, or perhaps the use of insulated foam pads for additional protection. Thermographic studies, using infrared detectors to measure heat loss, have shown that a particular test parka, under windchill tests, constructed with no zipper had a clo value of 2.04. With a zipper the clo value dropped to .93! Even more amazing was that the addition of a protected zipper cover and insulation tube increased the clo value to 2.17. Sewn-through seams particularly lower the clo value. Baffled construction avoids this problem, but adds thickness, weight, and expense to an item. A sewn-through construction is perfectly fine for clothing with lower clo value requirements, such as lightweight jackets, vests, etc.

A vacuum has the greatest insulation value of any material (or rather lack of it!) known. There is no conduction or convection loss of heat through a vacuum. Radiation loss still occurs but is curtailed by reflective insulation around the vacuum, the principle of the thermos bottle. However, reflective material is inefficient unless it is used in a vacuum (see page 34).

For practical purposes the best insulation we can obtain for clothing and sleeping gear is dry, still air. The warmed layer of air that surrounds a human has a clo value of .78! Convection currents easily strip this insulation layer away. Insulation materials such as down, Thinsulate, etc., will provide increased insulation because they stagnate or hold a thicker layer of air around the wearer. The less movement in this air, the better, since there is heat loss via convection currents.

A human's ability to leave a tropical climate to explore and populate the world was once dependent upon the development of protection from a hostile environment, and this was primarily accomplished with clothing. The use of animal skins, tanned with wood smoke and rubbing techniques, provided breathable, water-resistant, windproof insulation that, combined with various garment construction techniques, protected primitive humans from the elements. For centuries fabrics were constructed from natural plant fibers, animal hair, feathers, or fur augmented hides. The development of synthetic fibers, such as nylon or polyester, had a major technical and economic impact on clothing, tent, and sleeping bag construction for the modern outdoor traveler. Over the past few years improvements in these synthetic fibers have greatly increased our ability to protect ourselves.

Fiber and Fabric Construction

Cotton has been a mainstay of fabric construction since ancient times, but its use in outdoor clothing for temperature or cold climates cannot be condemned too highly. Designer and traditional brands of jeans have no place in the outdoors. Cotton allows heat to be conducted through it, even when dry, at a rate three times faster than wool, nylon, polyester, and acrylic fiber cloth. The latter four fibers are about equal in their dry insulation ability. Olefin (polypropylene) has about twice the dry insulation ability of those fibers and six times that of cotton. All manufacturers of outdoor clothing generally avoid pure cotton due to its poor insulation ability. Other major problems with cotton are its low evaporative ability and its very poor insulation ability when wet. Wet cotton allows thermal conductance to increase by a factor of nine, thus making it a danger to the wearer, unless you're in tropical conditions and want to bring about heat loss.

Cloth made of 65 percent Dacron with 35 percent cotton, however, provides strength, low cost, and rapid drying ability. Often referred to as "65-35 cloth," it is good material for work clothes and general outdoor wear, available at major chain retail stores. I have used it on my canoe trips with total satisfaction. It has actually been dry within a half hour after total immersion while being worn if the temperature is above 70°F (21°C) and the wearer is paddling a canoe or hiking at a moderate rate. I wear such a garment over polypropylene, or better yet polyester underwear, during winter travels.

Wool has been a proven outdoor protector for years. It can be woven into a thick, tight weave for optimal insulation ability. It can suspend water vapor within its fibers while retaining its insulating ability. Wool garments have a low wicking ability, which means that they are relatively dry even when wet. Fabrics made from wool are very wear resistant and moderately priced, but they are heavier than modern synthetics.

Synthetics like nylon, polyester, and acrylic evaporate water readily, are close to wool in insulation ability, but rapidly feel wet when damp. Nylon can be coated with different finishes to make excellent rain- and windproof garments or allowed to breathe without coatings. It is very durable, relatively inexpensive, and available in a variety of weights for different uses—from the very heavy duty cloth of backpacks to the lightweight ripstop nylon cloth used in sleeping bags and other breathable garments.

Olefin, or polypropylene, has been used in plastic sandwich bags for years. The production of a woven cloth from polypropylene fibers called *polypro* has proven valuable in the construction of underwear—either in net, lightweight weave, or heavy-duty bulk weave. This cloth has a great thermal insulation ability, almost twice that of wool. Thermal conductance measurements in kilocalorie/ square meter, polypro has a value of 1.2 compared to 2.1 for wool, 2.4 for nylon and most other synthetics, and the rather poor 6.1 of cotton. Its strong wicking ability allows it to remove moisture from the skin and transfer it to outer garments. It evaporates rapidly and will not readily feel damp. Polypro underwear is a great advantage to active outdoor sports enthusiasts. It is particularly useful for those activities requiring tremendous bursts of physical activity that often result in sweating, such as cross-country ski racing. Polypro's main disadvantage is that it retains body odors, even with cleaning.

Polyester pile garments are used for insulation as outer layers in spring/fall and middle layer insulation in winter clothing ensembles. As its fibers do not absorb water easily, these garments stay relatively dry and retain their insulation ability even if damp. The cost of these garments has decreased dramatically in the last few years, but they still tend to run toward expensive in price. They are extremely comfortable to wear and initially have the feel of soft bunny fur. They wear well for several major trips, but even the best-quality pile garments tend to become fuzzy or ragged after continual use and washings.

The greatest natural insulation batting is eider down. Its high loft per unit of weight results in considerable air trapping—the basis of clothing insulation—with very little garment weight. As it is highly compressible, bulky parkas and sleeping bags made with down will compress readily into small packages for ease in transportation when not in use. Frequently, pure down is augmented with a small percentage of feathers. This cuts the cost of the down mixture, but it also helps spring the down back into loft after it has been compressed. A major problem with down is its virtual total loss of insulation when wet. It is also expensive and in limited supply, most of it coming from mainland China.

Quallofil, PolarGard, and Hollofil II are examples of several synthetic fibers that have been developed especially for use as insulation batting. Their performance is far superior to cotton and wool batting. These fibers resist matting or clumping, they drain water off when wet, and still provide some thermal resistance when damp. They also have a high loft for their unit of weight. High loft fibers do not compress extremely well, but this can be an advantage; for example, a person sleeping on a mat of these materials in a sleeping bag will not decrease its insulation capability with her body weight. They are less expensive than down or high-grade feather mixtures.

Bulky insulated garments produce fewer problems with the bellows effect, or drafts, because of their form-fitting nature. If sewn with a quilting technique, however, they lose considerable insulation capability from compression at the seams. This can be eliminated with more costly sewing methods, such as internal baffling, which prevents the loft from sliding to the bottom of the garment, or by trapping the fill-in tubes that can then be covered with inner and outer layers of cloth, or sewn as double layers of tubes.

Microfilaments, another recent development, are manufactured to produce very thin mats of insulation that still yield considerable insulation. Brand names in U.S. markets include 3M's Thinsulate, DuPont's Sontique, and Eastman Chemical's KodOlite. The filaments of Thinsulate and Sontique are one-fifth the diameter of Hollofil or PolarGard, 4.5 microns in diameter compared to 25 microns. These microfilaments have about 2.1 times the insulation ability of an equal thickness of the older synthetic fiberfills. Such superior insulation with less thickness is due to better air trapping by their small fibers. These fibers literally allow air to cling to them (just as the larger fibers do). But with more fibers per unit of volume, the amount of air trapped, and therefore the insulation or thermal resistance value, is greater. Like the large fibers they do not retain water and provide excellent insulation when wet. While they provide about twice the insulating value of the other fiberfills per unit of thickness, their denser structure means they weigh 30 to 40 percent more per unit of thickness. This increased density will not allow the fabric to compress well into stuff sacks for carrying or storage, but makes it ideal in the construction of smaller insulated garments, like gloves.

There seems to be no limit to the improvement of special coatings and weaving techniques for these fibers. My current favorite is the Schoeller Textil "Dryskin" (www.schoeller-textiles.com) fabric, which combines abrasion resistance and windproofing with breathability and superior wicking capability.

Phase change technology has added a new dimension to fabric design. It consists of ways to impregnate a cloth with a substance that can turn from a crystal to a fluid state and remain in the fabric. Due to the latent heat of crystallization, energy is consumed during the melting phase and the wearer will feel cool. During the fluid melting phase, heat is released and the wearer feels warmth. This technique can enable "smart" cloth to cool you while you are active (storing heat) and then warm you while you are sitting still (releasing heat). As this technology improves, it will bring about significant changes in garment construction.

As mentioned above, many synthetic fibers maintain their thermal resistance rather well when damp. The accumulation of water weight still acts as a heat sump due to the physical nature of evaporation, which consumes large quantities of heat as described on page 14. For this reason, the old Inuit adage that "to sweat is to die" still holds true. The most crucial step to survival in a cold environment is to remain dry. This applies to the wearers of the new fabrics as much as the wearers of the traditional natural products of the past.

Breathable Fabrics versus Vapor Barrier

Centuries of outdoor activities have demonstrated the advisability of wearing breathable fabrics in cold weather. They allow the passage of water vapor from the skin to the outside atmosphere and minimize the amount of water that might otherwise be absorbed by the wearer's clothing.

A problem with breathable outer fabrics is that they also leak water from rain, drizzle, and melting snow or sleet. This can be minimized with the use of waterproof outer covers. However, insensible moisture loss through the skin, as well as possible sweating, can cause a considerable problem with moisture condensation on the interior surface of waterproof outer covers.

Insensible moisture loss is the water that leaves the skin by diffusion at the rate of 10 ounces (300 ml) per day. Frequently it pays not to wear an outer waterproof cover under conditions of light drizzle, as the amount of water that condenses on the inside of these jackets is considerably more than that provided by the inclement weather.

Ideally, an outer garment should be made from a material that is windproof, water repellent, and breathable. Several attempts have been made to approach this ideal. Coatings have been developed for breathable cloths, such as canvas and cordura nylon, which increase their water-repellent nature while maintaining their breathability. Special knitting techniques to provide this combination resulted in the production of Bulkflex and other materials. But the real breakthrough has come with the introduction of a micro-pore filter, protected by lamination and inserted between breathable, wearable, resistant fabrics.

Water molecules coalesce into particles. The micro-pore layer allows the passage of water vapor from the body because the layer's pores are about 700 times larger than a water molecule. Water from the atmosphere, even in its finest sprays, is a particulate clumping of hundreds of thousands of molecules that cannot pass through the micro-pore membrane. It is essential, of course, that these delicate micro-pore membranes be protected with a laminate that breathes very well. The major micro-pore fabrics in use today are Gore-Tex, Stomshed, and Klimate. Extensive personal use with these fabrics has demonstrated to me that they work well but can deteriorate with continual hard use. Our parkas were used on a daily basis for two years or more before failure, so the relative cost compared to the amount of use is quite reasonable. Investing in them is worthwhile for serious backcountry travelers and dwellers.

In the mid-1970s an aeronautical engineer, Jack Stephanson, popularized a new approach to outdoor wear—the *vapor barrier system*. This represented a 180 degree turn for the well-proven, breathable-layer principle. Proponents of the vapor barrier feel that it has two advantages. One is a decrease in dehydration and the other is the absolute protection of insulation from body moisture.

According to vapor barrier advocates, the insensible moisture loss of the skin can be decreased by ensuring a 100 percent layer of humidity on the surface. Insensible water loss is estimated to be about 37 ounces (1100 ml) per day, divided between respiration (which differs based on rate of breathing and the atmospheric temperature and humidity) and skin diffusion (a fairly steady 300 ml/day). While sweating is an active process used by the body to control overheating, insensible skin moisture is diffusion of moisture through interstitial cell spaces to outer skin layers. If this outer skin layer is dry, water continues to diffuse; if it is kept moist, however, it is thought that the diffusion process literally stops.

Trying to determine if this system works, as its advocates state, is very difficult. A review of the physiology literature fails to provide much help. While camping for up to thirteen days at temperatures at -20°F (-28°C) or below, I have found the use of a vapor barrier liner in my sleeping bag is a tremendous help. Without the liners the bags rapidly gain moisture, which freezes beneath the bag surface at a *freeze layer*—the point at which the temperature is at the freezing point that will exist between the warm interior and the below freezing exterior. This freeze layer builds a mantle of ice that continues to trap all further water passed through the skin. The ice shell provides some protection from the exterior bitter cold temperatures, even though the value of the original sleeping bag material has been decreased considerably by this wetting process. Sleeping in these solidly frozen bags is not comfortable, but at this point one is generally worried about survival, not comfort. These bags become extremely heavy and if rolled or stuffed into sacks in the morning, unrolling them is impossible the next night. The weight that these bags acquire is a direct reflection of the insensible moisture loss of the body during the period of time that they are used. The only exception would be additional water loss from respiration if one were to breath snuggled inside the bags, a technique that should be avoided.

Sir Charles Wright, a member of the second Scott expedition to the South Pole in 1910, related the problem they had with terrible sleeping bags icing during the trip: "When it was cold the bags just filled with ice and that was that. It took an hour to get in. Put your feet in. Melt that much. Shove further."

Their sleeping bags gained 30 pounds (13 kilograms) of ice. Since they could not be rolled in the morning they were loaded onto the sledges flat, with clothing stuffed into the openings to provide starting wedges, for getting back into them at night.

When using vapor barrier liners in our sleeping bags, we found very little moisture formation inside these liners, but the moisture may have escaped from the mouth of the bag. Also wearing polypro underwear makes sleeping in vapor barrier pleasant, once the initial warm-up period of about two minutes has passed. Climbing into a plastic bag at colder than -20°F (-30°C) is a thrill that anyone can do without, but it certainly proves well worth this effort, for crawling into a solidly frozen bag is much more difficult.

Some experts—or advertisers—have advised using vapor barrier during bitter cold weather as an undergarment during the day. Tight-fitting, waterproof jackets and pants, it is claimed, protect outer clothing from body moisture and decreased dehydration. A serious drawback with this, however, is ventilation of heat. Most work done under bitter winter conditions requires the expenditure of energy with sometimes a considerable amount of heat being generated, as indicated elsewhere in this book. While a vapor barrier will prevent sweat from wetting clothing, it is important to avoid overheating. Sweat must evaporate to help dissipate heat, which the vapor barrier will prevent. However, simply opening parkas and increasing exposure to bitter cold air will allow this heat dissipation. Outer garments, such as parkas, usually do not become damp from insensible moisture as the moisture is lost through the bellows effect. The *bellows effect* is caused by movement and by the amount of heat generated during the day. This produces a thermal drive that shoves moisture clear through the ensemble to freeze and evaporate or sublime off the surface, rather than forming an icy shell as occurs during bitter cold temperatures in sleeping bags.

I doubt that there is a decrease in dehydration from the daytime use of a vapor barrier under work clothes. Under bitter cold conditions the loss of water through respiration is greatly increased, far beyond the normal percentage of its usual contribution to insensible moisture loss. Especially with heavy exercise, the moisture loss through respiration will negate the slight saving afforded by the vapor barrier, which, at most, could amount to only 10 ounces (300 ml) per day. I do not believe that undergarment vapor barrier is a useful technology.

However, the use of a vapor barrier liner in boot socks works extremely well. It preserves outer socks from foot moisture, thus preserving their insulation ability. It is particularly important in protecting felt bootliners. I find it ideal to wear a pair of olefin wicking socks under a vapor barrier sock, and over that one or two pairs of heavy wool socks. Boots should be large enough to accommodate these layers without cramping the feet. Constriction of blood flow must be avoided under bitter cold conditions to help prevent frostbite.

The major manufacturers of vapor barrier liners currently are Stephensons Warmlite Equipment (RFD 4, Box 145, Briarcliff Avenue, Gilford, NH 03246) and Black Diamond, whose products are available at mountaineering specialty stores and catalogs. These items can be homemade from waterproofed nylon.

Dressing for Comfort versus Heat Conservation

Dr. William Kaufman at the University of Wisconsin, Green Bay has performed significant studies demonstrating that dressing for comfort may not provide proper protection from hypothermic environmental conditions. His work indicates that skin kept too warm would fail to allow various reflex actions to take place, thus lulling the body into a false sense of environmental security and allowing a core temperature drop to occur. This is in keeping with the concept of warm skin temperatures affecting the thermal set-point as described on page 50. His experiments do not indicate a profound drop, but the drop of 3.6°F (2°C) indicates a lack of proper energy conservation.

Figure 3-2 illustrates results from the above experiments. Individuals were dressed in a clothing ensemble that was rated for -26°F (-32°C) exposure. When exposed to that temperature, the core temperature remained fairly steady and generally rose about 0.9°F (0.5°C). When exposed to a temperature lower than the clothing was designed to handle, the core temperature initially rose as vasoconstriction and then shivering attempted to maintain the core temperature level. But the heat loss caused the core temperature to start falling, which it continued to do throughout the duration of the experiment. Surprisingly, upon exposure to a warmer temperature of -14.8°F (-26°C), the core temperature actually fell during the first 150 minutes, before returning to baseline levels. This illustrated the lack of thermoregulation on the part of the body when the skin was too warmly dressed, resulting in core temperature depression. Once the body caught on to the heat loss through significant core cooling, which exceeded the lowered thermal set-point, central temperature receptors caused the core temperature depression to be corrected.

Most outdoor travelers know that feeling a little coolness on the extremities is not unpleasant. This is a reason why an insulated vest makes such a comfortable addition to your outdoor clothing wardrobe. By keeping the torso warm and allowing the arms to cool, the body senses cold weather stress and adequately compensates to keep the core temperature from falling. The loss of energy stores might be insignificant for short-term exposure, and for long-term exposure the eventual correction of body thermal reflexes will apparently prevent a continued loss. These results might be most significant for repeated short-term exposure to the cold, say, leaving and entering a warm work area or cabin, which

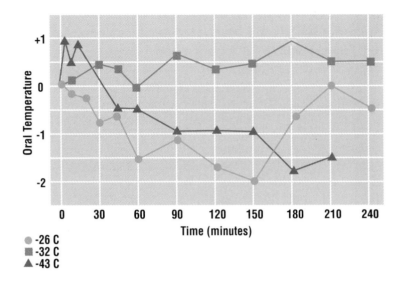

Figure 3-2

Core Temperature Drop from Improper Insulation

Changes in body sublingual temperature when dressed in clothing rated for −25.6°F (−32°C) and exposed to higher, equivalent, and lower environmental temperatures. Note that when exposed to a higher temperature (−14.8°F or −26°C), the core readings dropped during the first 150 minutes before returning to baseline at 210 minutes. This is probably due to the warm clothing fooling the thermoregulation mechanism, thus allowing unnecessary core heat loss.

(Adapted from W.C. Kaufman, "Cold Weather Clothing for Comfort or Heat Conservation," *Physician and Sportsmedicine*, February 1982.)

might fool the body into repeatedly failing to provide adequate thermal protection. It has been shown that repeated exposures to cold water and then rapid rewarming will cause a more pronounced drop in core temperature during the cold exposures than would otherwise be experienced.

The old woodsman's advice to dress comfortably cool when preparing for winter activity is proven by the above research. Certainly, if you are going to repeatedly expose yourself for short times to a cold environment, dress so that your trunk is warm, and your arms, hands, legs, and feet are somewhat cold.

Metallized Plastic Sheets:
Their Role and Limitations for Survival and Rescue

The cryogenics industries and the space research activities of NASA resulted in the development of aluminized plastic sheets, or *space blankets*. These have proven invaluable in the vacuum of space where radiation is the most important aspect of heat exchange. The use of metallized materials has been explored for possible use in the construction of warmer sleeping bags, gloves, and in the production of single- and double-layer sheets of coated plastic for use in survival situations.

The use of a sheet of any material has profound disadvantages in the wind. Wind tunnel experiments demonstrate that winds above 20 mph (32 km/hr) make sheeted materials unmanageable. Wrapping a patient in that wind speed can be accomplished only with extreme difficulty. The flapping soon produces gaps in the protection, and the wind rapidly carries away the entire sheet. Bags taped together from lightweight metallic plastic sheeting were more manageable, but at wind speeds above 20 mph they quickly disintegrated. Bags constructed from polyethylene of .12 mm thickness or greater and ripstop nylon could withstand winds of 40 mph (64 km/hr), even when intentionally punctured.

A Royal Air Force (UK) study on infrared reflection and heat conservation with metallized plastic sheeting failed to demonstrate any significant difference between using the reflective materials or plain plastic sheeting or ripstop nylon material in their experiments! Half of their studies were performed at –13°F (–25°C) in still air and half at 17°F (–8°C) in a wind speed of 10 mph (16 km/hr). Skin temperatures of the eight subjects for each experiment were measured wearing winter clothing and lying at rest. Particularly at the lower temperature, hoarfrost rapidly accumulated on the inside of the plastic sheeting, which effectively blocked the radiant reflective characteristics of the metallized surface.

The above study also demonstrates the reduction of a reflective material's ability to return radiant energy to the wearer when that material was woven into or layered within other material. A reflective heat barrier can provide only minor help when incorporated into clothing and sleeping gear. Sleeping gear and parkas that incorporate a reflective barrier in their design are not increasing the insulating ability significantly with this material, as the coated surface will not reflect as indicated in the experiments mentioned above. In fact, one might worry about the increased conduction that metal construction might cause. Reflective metallized ground covers are a particularly good example of this increased conduction. Plastic sheeting over foam is a better choice for a ground cover.

While providing virtually no radiation conservation at very cold temperatures, a metallized or plain plastic sheet can serve to protect from convection losses, up to the speed of its vulnerability to flapping or wind destruction. It also protects from the latent heat of evaporation losses. But it provides no protection from conduction loss, which in a hypothermia victim can be a very important source of heat loss, due to his increased surface area in contact with the ground or other cold surface.

Nutritional Requirements and Nonmuscular Heat Production

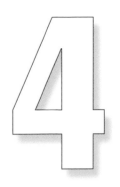

H eat is produced as a by-product of the metabolism required by cells to survive. The amount of metabolic heat produced by various organ systems differs, as can be seen in Figure 4-1. This *basal metabolic rate* (BMR) differs by age, sex, and at times by race and exposure to cold or heat stress. The BMR range is 40 to 60 kcal (170 to 250 kJ) per square meter body surface area. The average adult male body has 1.8 square meters of surface area.

The various organ systems produce about 72 percent of the basal metabolic heat when at rest, but only contribute approximately 25 percent of total heat production during exercise. The BMR produces about 70 kcal (290 kJ) per hour for the average weight (155 pound or 70 kilogram) man. Under conditions of cold stress the BMR can be increased by approximately 25 percent. This is probably effected by the release of a thyroid stimulating hormone, which increases the amount of the two active thyroid hormones in circulation, and by the increase in adrenal release of epinephrine and norepinephrine (adrenalin and noradrenalin).

The latter may cause increased utilization of "brown fat." It has been known that brown fat differs from normal fat or adipose tissue, which is a storage form of energy containing triglycerides and fatty acids. Brown fat is present in rodents and human infants; its presence in adults is now being studied. It appears to play a role in generating heat. Heat produced by this means is termed "nonshivering thermogenesis." The total amount of heat produced in this fashion is minimal when compared to the amount of heat produced by volitional

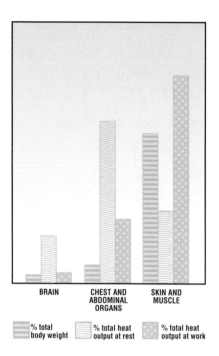

BRAIN	CHEST AND ABDOMINAL ORGANS	SKIN AND MUSCLE

% total body weight   % total heat output at rest   % total heat output at work

Figure 4-1

Percent of Heat Production versus Weight of Various Body Tissues During Work

This figure illustrates the percentage of body weight versus the amount of heat an organ produces in the working individual. The brain composes 2% of body weight, produces 16% of body heat production when at rest, but this drops to 3% of total body heat in the working subject. The chest and abdominal organs are 6% of body weight, produce 56% of body heat at rest, but only 22% of total heat output in the working individual. Skin and muscle are 52% of the total body weight, produce 18% of heat output in a resting subject, but can produce 25% to 73% of heat production in a resting person.

Adapted from Auerbach and Geehr, *Management of Wilderness and Environmental Emergencies*, Macmillan, 1983, and Selkurt *Physiology*, 4th Ed, 1976.

work and shivering, but it probably plays a role in the increased basal heat production noted during cold acclimatization.

The old saying, "we are what we eat," can be modified to "eat for heat." The source of metabolic and work-generated heat is the energy locked in the carbohydrate, fat, and protein that we consume. These three nutrients supply the calories. It is important to obtain not only an adequate total number of calories per day based on expected requirements, but also a proper mix of these three nutrients should be consumed to derive the maximum benefit. This has a particular value with weight conscious backpackers who wish to obtain the most benefit for the least weight.

Nutritional Sources of Heat Production

Carbohydrates

Carbohydrates consist of starches and sugars that are broken down into simple sugars called monosaccharides. The latter are absorbed from the intestines and transported directly to the liver by a closed circulatory system known as the portal system. The liver is responsible for maintaining a nearly constant supply of monosaccharide "glucose" in the blood at all times. When glucose is absorbed after a meal or a candy tablet is digested, the liver quickly converts it to glycogen. In turn, glycogen can be broken down into glucose during periods of fasting (which includes any period during which no food is being digested). During rest, muscle tissue also forms glycogen, rather slowly, from the glucose liberated by the liver into the general systemic circulation, which is then stored in the muscle to be consumed during active periods.

As all carbohydrates are converted into glucose before being utilized by the body for energy, it makes no difference which of the various forms of carbohydrate are consumed. Starches take a little longer to digest and be absorbed in an experimental model in which the stomach is empty and glucose solution is compared to starch solution during uptake experiments. But in a human with food in the intestines, this starch will be broken down into sugars (monosaccharides) by the time the absorptive position in the intestines is reached, and any difference in the rate of uptake between complex starches and pure glucose will be of no practical value.

One gram of carbohydrate produces 4 kcal (17 kJ) of energy. This actually varies from 4.2 kcal (17.6 kJ) per gram of starch to 3.7 kcal (15.5 kJ) per gram of glucose, but the average used in dietetic computations is 4 kcal per gram of carbohydrate. The liver has a limited storage capacity for glycogen and when this excess is reached, the adipose, or fat-forming tissue of the body, does just what its name indicates—it forms fat. Usually 50 percent or more of the diet is supplied by carbohydrates. Carbohydrate intake is often the principle variable in weight loss or gain. A minimum of 5 grams (or 20 kcal) of carbohydrate per 100 kcal of total diet is required to prevent a condition known as ketosis (which results from the metabolism of fat components called "fatty acids" exclusively).

As mentioned above, the rapidity of uptake of sugar is not subject to tremendous changes in a human due to the type of sugar or starch, or even to the type of other fluid or food components with which it is consumed. There are many products on the market that claim they will replace blood sugar more rapidly than a regular sucrose tablet. This change in rapidity of uptake is minimal. In fact, the rapidity of uptake of sucrose over the more complex forms of carbohydrate, the starches, is virtually insignificant.

In other words, there is no quick way to get sugar into the bloodstream by mouth that does a much better job than a candy bar.

The next shocker for many people is that once this sugar is in the bloodstream, *it is not available for instant energy.* Many athletes, hikers, runners, and others will remark on how a candy bar provided them a quick energy pickup and that an "emergency energy lift" can and should be provided by carrying candy tablets or bars while hiking, etc.

The return of blood glucose levels to normal has a positive effect on the brain, which exclusively must rely on glucose for metabolism. This feeling of well-being is very helpful for mental function, but to assimilate the glucose into actual energy takes both food and rest. The rate at which we can turn food into energy is age dependent and, most particularly, dependent upon the level of our physical conditioning.

Eating a high-energy carbohydrate snack does not provide instant energy substrates that will aid increasing exercise tolerance. The only method of increasing this tolerance is pretrip exercise or training. Training causes an increase in the ability of the cells' enzyme systems to process glucose into muscle glycogen and to utilize this glycogen in producing work or heat energy. There is no easy way around training one's body for work. Eating a candy bar hoping for some free and easy burst of energy will not provide an instant ability to do work or produce heat.

It is necessary to consume food substrates to replace the energy that we have consumed through exercise and heat production. While carbohydrates have gotten much of the publicity and study since glucose (a carbohydrate) is an immediate precursor of the high energy substrates, fat and protein are also essential in this process and must be consumed in adequate quantity.

Protein

Shortly after the Persian Wars, an athlete and trainer, Dromeus of Stymphalus, winner of the long race at Olympia in 460 and 456 B.C., introduced the high protein meat diet. It was erroneously felt that during heavy exercise large losses of protein would be encountered.

This attitude about the necessity of a high protein diet has persisted among many athletes, but the following should be noted: (1) Protein is not an efficient energy fuel; (2) The body does not store protein in the sense that it stores fat; (3) Excess protein does not increase strength; and (4) It often takes greater energy to metabolize and digest protein. Protein intake requirements differ by age, size, and sex.

However, with regard to protein we are interested in *quality* as well as *quantity*. Our muscle structure is composed of protein. Protein, during starvation periods, can also be converted to energy. Obviously this is to be avoided as it leads to a decrease in strength. It actually provides an inferior source of energy as it provides only 4 kcal (17 kJ) of energy per gram, with considerable wastage during its processing (see "Specific Dynamic Action of Food" below).

Proteins consist of building blocks called amino acids. Approximately twenty different amino acids make up the proteins in our bodies. These amino acids are interchangeable—all, that is, except for eight amino acids that cannot be synthesized by humans. It is important that these eight amino acids be included in our diet, as it will be the only way we have of acquiring them for incorporation. Protein foods of animal origin contain these essential eight amino acids in nearly optimal amounts and are thus said to be "high-quality proteins." Only a carefully selected balance of various non-meat proteins can provide proper ratios of the eight essential amino acids. Strict vegetarians should consult a physician or a registered dietitian for proper advice on this matter.

Fat

How about a nice slice of blubber? Sounds rather repulsive to our civilized ears, doesn't it? And too bad, since fats have a very high energy value, more than twice the energy per weight of carbohydrate or protein. Many studies show no indication of fat hunger or craving due to cold stress. This, however, overlooks the very point made by the great Arctic explorer, Vilhjalmus Stefansson: that is, a high fat diet was the basis of survival of the Inuit (Eskimo). Due to the inadequate intake of fat, western expedition after expedition dies of exposure in the same area that was tolerated by entire families of Inuit. The turning point of High Arctic exploration was made by those explorers who emulated the Inuit diet. But in the modern literature this discovery is being lost. It was an expensive lesson in the past. In studying the journals of many of these disasters, the turning point seems to occur after the first debilitating year in the field. This indicates that while it is not critical to increase the fat content of trips lasting shorter periods of time to cold areas, a higher fat diet has many qualities that support its use. The significant exception is during high altitude trips, as indicated below in the section on winter energy requirements.

Fats have a calculated food value of 9.45 kcal (40 kJ) per gram. For rough calculations, the value 9 kcal per gram is used, thus including a realistic 5 percent loss in the efficiency of digestion and absorption from the intestines.

Specific Dynamic Action of Food

These nutrients not only allow the formation of heat through the work the muscle can perform consuming muscle glycogen, but their very assimilation by the body produces heat. This amounts to a processing energy cost called the *specific dynamic action of food* (SDA), also called the *thermic effect of food* (TE) or *diet-induced thermogenesis* (DIT). In other words, the body must expend energy to metabolize these nutrients. And this energy results in heat.

The *thermic effect of food* also pertains to other aspects of nutrition and heat production. Defined as "the increase in metabolic rate after ingestion of a meal," it was shown in early 1980 that alcohol, tea, and coffee significantly increase the metabolic rate. One of the most interesting studies is titled "Effect of Spiced Food on Metabolic Rate" by C.I. Henry and B. Emery, published in March 1986 in *Human Nutrition*. They demonstrated that chile (red pepper, *Capsicum annum*) and mustard (*Brassica juncea*) also increased the metabolic rate. From practical experience I know that these effects vary from individual to individual. Some people break out in a profuse sweat when eating hot peppers, while others do not. The late Sandy Bridges, formerly with the BSA Northern Tier High Adventure Base, one of the world's leading authorities on cold weather camping, refused hot coffee in camp at night as it made him sweat. As the golden rule of winter camping is never to perspire, coffee was not on his provision list! I, on the other hand, find that coffee, tea, and certainly hot pepper sauces (I prefer habañero peppers) are perfect for the trail. There is some concern that coffee and tea are diuretics and will lead to dehydration. I do not believe that the diuretic effect is very large, but I am convinced of their significant thermic effect.

The SDA of food is expressed in the number of kcal required to metabolize that particular nutrient or amount of food. Pure carbohydrates consume 5 percent of their value during their assimilation. Fats consume 13 percent and proteins 30 percent of their caloric value to be processed. Most of this energy is released as heat during the two hours after ingestion.

Energy can be spared and fewer calories eaten, if the basic nutrients are eaten in the proper proportions. That is to say, the specific dynamic action of food is reduced (i.e., the amount of energy wasted to process the food just ingested is reduced) when proper ratios of fat, carbohydrate, and protein are consumed. For example, a mixed diet of protein and carbohydrate consumes 12.5 percent less calories to process than predicted. A mixed diet of protein and fat consumes 54 percent less than predicted!

The percentage of fat in the diet, therefore, plays an important role in obtaining more efficiency from the weight of the food consumed. At amounts of up to 3,000 kcal (12,600 kJ), 20 to 25 percent of the total intake should be fat (66 to 83 grams of fat—about 2 ounces). At higher caloric values, 30 to 35 percent should probably come from fat. Of the total grams of fat in the diet, 1 percent should consist of polyunsaturated oil in order to include the essential fatty linoleic and arachidonic acids which aid in proper fat metabolism.

The higher caloric requirements of winter camping can be easily met by increasing fat content of meals by adding cooking oil. This may be added to pancake batter and stews without being noticeable, even by those who do not like fats. The use of butter also makes a palatable addition to the diet.

Winter Energy Requirements

Energy loss is controlled during exposure to cold temperatures by wearing insulation (clothing), but an increase in total kcal requirement is expected depending on the type of activity (many winter projects are physically difficult) and the extra weights of winter clothing. In calculating nutritional requirements for winter camping I have found that our daily consumption was never over 4,200 kcal (17,600 kJ). Frequently it was around 3,700 kcal (15,500 kJ). I have developed these figures both by noting what was consumed during many winter trips into northern Canada and by calculating theoretical energy requirements for work and basal metabolism. Jack Drury, a former president of the Wilderness Education Association and consultant on high adventure outdoor activities, calculates a maximal requirement of 4,200 kcal (17,600 kJ) per day as the nutritional requirement for his college students during strenuous winter expeditions in the Adirondacks.

One frequently reads that a winter camping diet will require 6,000 kcal (25,000 kJ). Very few people are physically conditioned to consume and utilize such an enormous load of food. It is true that conditioned lumberjacks or world class athletes require such massive amounts of calories, but generally in planning your winter trip, even to the Arctic, do not overload your budget or back with unnecessary calories.

While the higher calorie requirement of winter activity generally means that a larger percentage of fat should be included, there are certain exceptions. At high altitudes, particularly above 16,000 feet (4,877 meters), the fat content of the diet should be reduced due to a profound aversion for fats that develops at these elevations. Some persons are affected as low as 15,000 feet (4,572 meters). Conversely, sugar is well tolerated at high altitude with two to three times the normal amount being readily consumed in drinks. There is a craving for fresh meat, or highly spiced meat, rather than tinned or freeze-dried foods. But at high altitude it appears that carbohydrates win the taste test over both protein and fat.

Water

Hydration, or adequate water intake, is extremely important. Natick Army Laboratories have found that a 10 percent dehydration will cause a 30 to 40 percent decrease in thermal control. Our water requirements include 800 to 1,000 ml in the urine, 100 ml in stool, and 600 to 1,000 ml as insensible loss through our lungs and skin for a total daily requirement of a minimum of 1,500 ml (1.6 qts.).

A factor predisposing an individual to dehydration is the dry relative humidity under cold weather conditions. All air must be warmed to approximately core temperature and moisture content of this heated air raised to nearly 100 percent humidity during respiration. If a person is active under these cold, dry conditions, the amount of moisture lost through respiration increases and must be replaced. It is essential to keep up with this loss, with frequent replacement during the day on an hourly basis, if possible.

Thirst lags behind actual water requirements, so water loss must be anticipated and fluid taken before thirst occurs. A useful winter method of ensuring adequate fluid intake is to notice the color of the urine in snow. If it becomes dark and yellow-orange, it is becoming too concentrated and indicates inadequate water intake. It appears that a daily intake of three liters of water will provide adequate protection from dehydration for most activities under cold stress conditions.

A liter (1.05 quarts) heated to 130°F (55°C), about as warm as most people can drink, would provide approximately 18 kcal (75 kJ) of heat to a normothermic individual. A liter of water at the freezing point would absorb 37 kcal (155 kJ) of energy to heat it to normal core temperature. It is obvious that very warm water cannot replace very many calories, while very cold water can leach a certain number of calories away. There is a thirst-quenching aspect of cold water that makes most cold weather travelers crave it. With adequate heat production, the intake of cold water will do no harm. In a hypothermic individual, it would be best to avoid a further calorie drain, but if the choice is between cold water or no water, give the cold water. The rescuer could warm the water with his own body heat to minimize the heat loss, but this heat loss is minimal while the dehydration aspect of this problem is of maximal concern.

We have frequently been warned not to eat snow due to its cooling effect and the harm that it might do us while traveling under cold stress conditions. Popular stories tell us that eating snow is as bad for us as drinking seawater. Snow will leach additional heat from us. The temperature of the snow must be considered, for surface snow will be as cold as the local air temperature, while deeper snow will be as cold as the recent average temperature. If the weather has been –40°, a liter would require 77 kcal (323 kJ) of heat to bring it to normal body temperature and an additional 79.7 kcal (334 kJ) to melt the ice. This has become a substantial amount of heat loss, in fact 157 kcal (698 kJ). The additional heat consumption to actually melt the ice crystals to liquid water [79.71 kcal per kilogram or liter of water (2.2 pounds or 1.06 quarts)] is called the "latent heat of crystallization" or the "latent heat of fusion."

Snow can be consumed only if there is considerable heat production in a person with good nutrition, who is not fatigued. Snow at a temperature close to the melting point is safer than cold snow with regard to heat loss. Bitter cold snow could do damage by freezing the delicate tissues lining the oral cavity and throat. It is much safer to melt snow prior to consuming it. Adding snow to water already melted will avoid scorching the snow and will provide more water which, while cooler, will quench the thirst with minimal calorie loss.

You will occasionally read that eating snow will cause dehydration. There is no basis in fact for this statement.

Muscular Heat Production

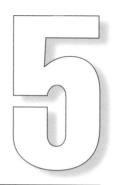

esides basal metabolic heat generation, the active controlled use of skeletal muscles is a primary method of generating heat. This is the heat produced by hiking, climbing, cutting wood—in general the purposeful engagement of any outdoor activity. As noted, the basal metabolic rate for the average 155 pound (70 kg) male is approximately 70 kcal per hour. This reflects a basal metabolic rate of 1,700 kcal per day. Skiing cross-country uphill at maximal speed on hard snow can generate 18 to 19 kcal/min (an awesome 1,100 kcal/hr), but this would only be possible for someone who was in world class competition condition, and then for only a limited time.

But even less conditioned individuals can increase their heat production significantly by purposeful exercise. A 180 pound man walking at 2 mph on a hard surface would use 210 kcal per hr; this work would increase to 828 kcal per hr in soft snow with snow shoes on, if he was able to walk 2.5 mph. Chopping firewood burns 294 kcal per hr during sustained activity. A man in good physical condition can sustain a work output up to 630 kcal per hr for long periods of time.

Thus purposeful exercise can not only accomplish an outdoor task, but it provides substantial heat. Table 5-1 demonstrates a variety of outdoor tasks and the amount of kcal of heat that these activities generate.

There are limitations to the amount of purposeful exercise that an individual can accomplish. Physical conditioning is the key, as exhaustion and the body's inability to continue muscular activity can readily result in hypothermia. The consumption of the energy substrate in the muscle, the muscle glycogen, is the end point of the ability to continue muscular activity. Physical conditioning increases the muscle's ability to replace this essential glycogen store and enhances its ability to utilize it.

Table 5-1
....

Gross Energy Costs for Different Activities of Average Young Adults (Multiply kcal by 4.19 to determine kJ)

	kcal/min.		kcal/min.
Sleep, resting	1.0–1.2	Running, cross country	
Sitting, at ease, resting	1.5	140 lb. subject	10.6
Sitting, writing, card play	2.1	Skiing	
Standing, at ease	1.7	level, hard snow, 4 mph	9–10
Dressing, washing	3.0–4.0	moderate speed	11–16
Walking, 2 mph, level, hard surface		uphill, hard snow, max speed	18–19
100 lb. subject	2.2	Climbing, slope 1 in 5.7 grade	
140 lb. subject	2.9	180 lb. subject	
160 lb. subject	3.2	with 11 lb. load	10.7
180 lb. subject[1]	3.5	with 22 lb. load	11.6
Walking, 3.5 mph, level, hard surface		with 44 lb. load	12.2
100 lb. subject	3.6	Climbing, slope 1 in 4.7 grade	
140 lb. subject[2]	4.6	180 lb. subject	
160 lb. subject	5.0	with 11 lb. load	12.1
180 lb. subject[3]	5.4	with 22 lb. load	12.7
Walking, 4 mph, level, hard surface		with 44 lb. load	13.2
100 lb. subject	4.1	Canoeing[6]	
140 lb. subject	5.2	2.5 mph	3.0
160 lb. subject	5.8	4.0 mph	7.0
180 lb. subject	6.4	Cycling[7]	
Walking, 4.5 mph, level, hard surface		5.5 mph	4.5
155 lb. subject[4]	7.2	9.4 mph	7.0
Walking, 5 mph, level, hard surface		13.1	11.1
155 lb. subject	10.5	Breaking firewood	4.9
Walking, 2 mph, up 15% incline		Driving a car	2.8
155 lb. subject[5]	7.5	Driving a motorcycle	3.4
Walking, 2 mph, up 25% incline		Volleyball	3.5
155 lb. subject	10.6	Tennis	7.1
Walking, 3 mph, up 5% incline		Swimming	
155 lb. subject	6.0	Backstroke	
Walking, 3 mph, up 10% incline		25 yd./min.	5.0
155 lb. subject	7.8	30 yd./min	7.0
Walking, 3 mph, up 15% incline		35 yd./min.	9.0
155 lb. subject	10.5	40 yd./min.	11.0
Walking, 3.5 mph, up 10% incline		Breast stroke	
155 lb. subject	8.9	40 yd./min.	10.0
		Side stroke	
		40 yd./min.	11.0

Note 1. At 2.5 mph a 180 lb. subject would increase work to 13.8 on soft snow with snow shoes, with 44 lb. load 20.2

Note 2. At 3.5 mph a 140 lb. subject would increase work to 5.7 on level grass, 6.2 on stubble field, 7 on ploughed field

Note 3. At 3.5 mph a 180 lb. subject would increase work to 11.9 on hard snow

Note 4. When markedly rough, slower speed will compensate for surface difference

Note 5. Walking down a 10% decline at various speeds will result in up to 25% less energy requirement than level surface; very steep decline will increase work above level surface—no figures available

Note 6. Canoe data for moderately skilled subjects, favorable weather, average of 4 trials for this data

Note 7. Wide tires add 1 kcal/min. for all speeds

Adapted from Passmore, R., and Durnin, J. V. G. A.: "Human Energy Expenditure," *Physiol. Rev.,* 35:801-840, 1955

Physical conditioning is of the utmost importance in preparing for cold stress. There is no easy way around it.

The Shiver Response

Another important method of thermogenesis, or heat formation, is shivering. This uncontrolled, rhythmic contraction/relaxation of skeletal muscle is an important emergency measure that the body has to prevent further core heat loss. It is initiated by a cold receptor located in the hypothalamus of the brain, but it also works with input from skin sensors, primarily located on the trunk of the body. This remarkable reflex activity causes antagonistic groups of muscle to oscillate at a frequency of six to twelve cycles per second.

In the hierarchy of maintaining body heat, shivering plays both important stop-gap and fine-tuning roles. If we have not provided adequate additional heat, if we have not added enough insulation to our clothing, if purposeful muscle activity has not provided adequate additional heat, and if the body's various heat preservation reflexes have not kept the core temperature above 97°F (36°C), shivering will result.

An initial shiver in a warm person may also result from sudden cooling of the skin or inhalation of cold air, thus providing a rapid warming function. This "early shiver response" helps establish other reflex mechanisms to protect the core temperature and does not represent a dropping core temperature.

Shivering can increase heat production from 2 to about 4.5 times the resting rate of heat production, resulting in an additional 200 to 500 kcal (838 to 2,100 kJ) per hour. But at a price. It is a highly inefficient method of heat production. While shivering, the body is willing to squander remaining energy stores, totally depleting muscle glycogen stores and energy substrates available to it in the desperate attempt to keep core temperature from falling further.

If core temperature remains depressed, shivering will continue. If the core temperature rises, shivering will stop. Shivering will also stop if the energy substrates "run out." At that point a precipitous drop in core temperature will occur. The violent shiver is the body's last serious defense against sliding into potentially lethal deep hypothermia.

Shivering plays an important role in rescuing hypothermic individuals. If they are able to shiver, they are capable of reheating themselves. Applying small amounts of heat to the skin's surface might prevent this response and actually decrease their rewarming rate. If they are unable to shiver, they are either too cold for their muscles to work or they are exhausted. These people are unable to reheat themselves spontaneously and will require the addition of heat to rewarm (see page 58).

In case of rapid heat loss, such as in cold water immersion hypothermia, depression of the core temperature can occur so quickly that shivering ceases even though energy substrates are still available. Evidence indicates that this suppression of the shiver reflex probably occurs at 86°F (30°C). it appears that alcohol suppresses the shiver reflex. The fact that these victims have not exhausted energy substrate stores may affect their ability to survive when they are reheated, although many other factors are also important when examining the differences between a slow onset or chronic hypothermia and a rapid onset, or acute immersion hypothermia.

Besides being an inefficient use of valuable energy stores, the shiver response causes an increased blood flow to muscles and therefore pulls blood from the body core. This increased circulation causes a loss of insulation and increases heat loss by about 25 percent. Of course, this loss is offset by the increased heat production of 200 to 500 percent as mentioned above.

A few other facts should be mentioned concerning the very valuable shiver response. First, some people do not have a shiver response, and in others the ability to shiver is diminished. And second, do not be overly afraid of shivering. It is a useful method of fine tuning the body heat production and it does not mean that one is in imminent danger of hypothermia. A greater danger than shivering is the feeling of exhaustion.

While shivering will rapidly lead to exhaustion, it is easy to see that an exhausted person will have lost the ability to shiver. Thus, exhaustion by itself strips away this valuable last-ditch defense mechanism of the body. In order to properly tolerate exposure to hypothermia conditions, we must strive *not* to become exhausted and *not* to have to rely on shivering to maintain our core temperature. We must use whatever intellect we have available to counter further heat loss and otherwise improve our chances of survival at this moment. A further decrease in core temperature will certainly occur when substrates have been exhausted. This core decrease will subsequently depress our mental ability to cope properly with the emergency situation.

We have been warned in the lore of the north not to dare stop and rest lest we fail to awaken and freeze to death. I traveled north once with a person who had just read *Call of the Wild.* It was virtually impossible to get that person to agree to a rest stop due to the fear of freezing to death. But maintaining a reserve of that precious muscle glycogen and minimizing the general level of fatigue are critical factors in assuring our survival in a cold stress situation. All of the factors causing fatigue are not fully understood, but it is without a doubt a warning of imminent exhaustion. This exhaustion must not be allowed to occur because with it we lose the ability to do work or to shiver—both of the major body functions that produce heat to prevent hypothermia. Only with adequate insulation can an exhausted person be protected from hypothermia.

In this book I have tackled two popular myths. First, that one should keep going, lest one freeze to death. The other, eat candy for instant energy for continued work and prevention of hypothermia. Scientific evidence demonstrates that both of these ideas are faulty. Rest is important. The cold-exposed individual should rest to prevent exhaustion and will need to seek adequate protection from the cold during the rest period. He should also eat to replace energy substrates. But it must be understood that energy acquired from eating will be slow in coming and its speed in replenishing muscle glycogen stores will be dependent upon prior physical conditioning. A sensible approach to enjoying a safe, prolonged exposure to hypothermic conditions is:

1. Proper pretrip physical conditioning

2. Proper pretrip nutritional status

3. Proper dress

4. Adequate rest during the trip

5. Adequate nutrition to replenish energy stores while on the trip

6. Adequate hydration while on the trip

Physiological Responses to Prevent Heat Loss

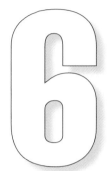

A warm blooded organism such as a human is scientifically termed a *homeotherm*. This is an organism that must maintain its body temperature within a narrow range (101° to 96°F or 38° to 35.5°C) to properly function. The organism internally generates heat to accomplish this. The environment can either aid or hinder this process by adding more heat or by sapping it away.

An environmental (ambient) temperature of less than 77°F (25°C) results in a lowering of the core temperature of a naked human, unless either a mental or physiological response to counter that drop occurs.

The Body Core Temperature Set-Point

To maintain the core temperature within this optimum range, the body reflexes must respond rapidly and accurately to conditions of increased or decreased environmental temperature and increased or decreased muscle activity. It does this by establishing a precise internal temperature set-point that is monitored by a portion of the brain, the hypothalamus. This set-point is usually at precisely 99.8°F (37.7°C).

As it turns out, the most significant way to change the core temperature set-point is to change the skin temperature. The body needs to anticipate a sudden transition into a hot or cold environment before the core blood temperature actually changes. However, it also does not want to overreact to local skin temperature and over-cool or overheat unnecessarily.

While skin will vasoconstrict and a local shiver response will occur upon local application of cold, a relatively normal core temperature set-point prevents a body-wide shiver reflex. If an increasing surface area of skin is cooled, generalized shivering will start at relatively

B A S I C   E S S E N T I A L S

normal core temperature as the set-point is changed to a lower level to respond to this threat of cooling.

The addition of heat to the skin surface during rescue could alter the set-point to a higher level, suppress shivering, and decrease vasoconstriction. Of course, if the patient is exhausted, there will be no ability to shiver anyway, and providing an appropriate amount of heat to this individual will be beneficial.

Vascular Control of Thermoregulation

An interesting aspect of body heat control is that 95 percent of the heat produced daily by the body must be removed. Yet under exposure to a cold environment a mechanism must be available to decrease this remarkable heat loss.

For thermoregulation purposes body heat is regulated in two zones: the inner core and the mantle regions. The inner core is constantly producing heat internally through the basal metabolic activity of the organ systems and the specific dynamic action of food. Muscle activity, located in the inner mantle region, also produces heat by contraction. The outer, or exterior, mantle region, consisting of the skin and subcutaneous fat layer, is where most of the process of heat elimination takes place.

Body fluids, fat, and muscle are good thermal insulators and poor conductors. A 0.4 inch (1 centimeter) thick piece of perfused muscle is as good an insulator as a thick piece of cork (conductivity = 18 kcal/hr/°C gradient). A man at rest produces about 72 kcal (300 kJ) of heat per hour. The amount of heat conductance from the core to the mantle will equal from 5 to 10 kcal per degree Celsius gradient per hour. With the amount of insulation present in his mantle, only 20 to 40 kcal per hour of heat could be transported to the surface, depending upon the temperature gradient. Internal heat cannot, therefore, be readily eliminated by conductance.

The majority of internal heat is eliminated by forced convection in which warm blood from the interior is carried to the cooler surface of the mantle by the circulation system. The skin has remarkable properties allowing extensive regulation of blood flow, both from local factors and central nervous system control. This blood flow can range from 30 ml/min (0.5 percent of cardiac output) under cold stress conditions, to 300 ml/min (5 percent of cardiac output) under normal temperature conditions, to 3,000 ml/min during times of high heat stress.

There are two major components in this change of blood flow that play enormous roles in the rate of heat transfer. One is vasoconstriction, the other vasodilation. The process of vasodilation can increase blood flow to the outer skin surface, the epidermis, by one hundredfold, thus increasing heat loss by as much as twentyfold. Similarly, vasoconstriction can effectively increase the insulting depth of the outer mantle by decreasing blood flow.

Linkages of surface blood veins and deep veins, which carry the peripheral blood back to the core, are responsible for considerable heat conservation. The deep veins travel in a neurovascular bundle, the importance of which is their close proximity to the artery carrying warmer blood outward to the extremity. Under cold stress there is a shift in venous blood from the outer veins to these inner veins. This allows a conductive heat exchange between the cool blood flowing back and the warm blood flowing outward. This is called the *countercurrent heat exchange*. Cool venous blood is warmed as it returns to the core, and arterial blood is cooled as it travels away from the core. Blood circulation to the extremities continues, while heat loss is minimized, since heat is not carried away by the flow. In times of heat stress, the returning venous blood is carried primarily in the surface veins and away from the warm arterial heat source, thus preventing the returning cooler blood from being heated by the hot arterial blood.

These vasoconstrictor and blood flow shifts are so effective that upon exposure to cold, a rise of the core temperature of 0.9°F (0.5°C) occurs. This change in circulation effectively increases the mantle depth and decreases the core size, thus protecting the core temperature but allowing the loss of some heat stores during cold response.

It is easy to glide over a statement such as "loss of some heat stores" without realizing its significance. This means that the total amount of heat in the body will be allowed to decrease as the mass of tissue in the smaller core attempts to remain warm and the mantle becomes larger and is allowed to become cooler. The body gives up trying to heat its entire mass and by simply maintaining the smaller interior core near normal temperature, the total amount of heat in the body (which can be computed by multiplying mass times temperature) has decreased. See Figure 6-1. This fact is particularly important in rescue work, when we need to consider the total amount of heat required to rewarm a victim, or in considering the amount of heat that a rescuer may be able to provide with her own body.

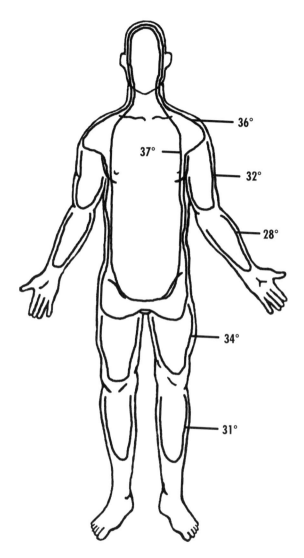

Figure 6-1

A Cold-Stressed Individual

As the body gets colder, the core temperature shrinks, leaving a larger, cooler mantle formation. This initially provides a greater insulation layer from cold, but it means a decreased total heat store.

Detection and Prevention of Chronic Hypothermia

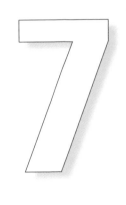

Detection of Chronic Hypothermia

The greatest single clue that a person can become a victim of chronic hypothermia is the development of exhaustion. An exhausted person will soon decrease her ability to produce heat. If she is not able to obtain protection from the cold when heat production decrease has occurred, her core temperature will cool. Watch for exhaustion. Recognizing exhaustion in a trip member provides the trip leader with a window of opportunity to make a decision that might save that member's life.

The person with a core temperature below 95°F (35°C) will begin developing the signs and symptoms of hypothermia. While no specific indications signal a particular core temperature, a general impression of core temperature can be deduced from the symptoms which the patient demonstrates as indicated in Table 7-1.

Do not rely on a symptom table too heavily, for hypothermia is notorious for the varying signs that different people exhibit. The single most useful clue that a person is suffering from mild hypothermia is the development of *ataxia*, a loss of coordination indicated, for example, by the inability to walk a 30-foot (9 meter) straight line. If a person is incapable of doing this, he is hypothermic, even if he denies it. Other possible reasons that might also result in ataxia could be high altitude cerebral edema (which requires descent for treatment) or drunkenness from alcohol or drug use (which requires rethinking about how to choose your travel companions). A

Table 7-1
....

Signs and Symptoms of Hypothermia

CORE TEMP	SIGNS AND SYMPTOMS
99° to 97°F (37°C to 36°C)	Normal temperature range; shivering may begin
97° to 95°F (36°C to 35°C)	Cold sensation, goose bumps, unable to perform complex tasks with hands, shivering can be mild to severe, skin numb
95° to 93°F (35°C to 34°C)	Shivering intense, muscle incoordination becomes apparent, movements slow and labored, stumbling pace, mild confusion, may appear alert. *Best field test for hypothermia:* inability to walk a 30-ft. line properly
93° to 90°F (34°C to 32°C)	Violent shivering persists. difficulty speaking, sluggish thinking, amnesia starts to appear and may retrograde, gross muscle movements sluggish, unable to use hands, stumbles frequently, difficulty speaking, signs of depression
90° to 86°F (32°C to 30°C)	Shivering stops in chronic hypothermia, exposed skin blue or puffy, muscle coordination very poor with inability to walk, confusion, incoherent, irrational behavior, *but may be able to maintain posture and appearance of psychological contact*
86° to 82°F (30°C to 27.7°C)	Muscles severely rigid, semiconscious, stupor, loss of psychological contact, pulse and respirations slow, pupils can dilate
82° to 78°F (27.7°C to 25.5°C)	Unconsciousness, heartbeat and respiration erratic, pulse and heartbeat may be inapparent, muscle tendon reflexes cease
78° to 75°F (25.5°C to 24°C)	Pulmonary edema, failure of cardiac and respiratory centers, probable death. *Death may occur before this level.*
59° (15.2°C)	Lowest recorded temperature of chronic hypothermia survivor, Japan, reported 1986
48.2°F (9°C)	Lowest recorded temperature of induced hypothermia in surgical patient with survival, 1958

person who cannot stand is probably suffering from profound chronic hypothermia and must be treated as such.

Prevention of Chronic Hypothermia

There are a variety of intellectual responses appropriate during exposure to cold weather that minimize the chances of developing hypothermia.

When Active, Ventilate Excess Heat

It is perfectly proper, in fact necessary, to ventilate excess heat to the environment. If your activity level is high enough to produce sweating, it must be avoided by allowing cold air contact with the underlayers of your winter outfit, or even with your skin. This will require opening parkas, removing mittens, taking your hat off, or whatever is necessary to prevent overheating.

When Tired, Preserve Energy

When you feel exhaustion developing, or otherwise know that your physical limitations are being reached, it will be necessary to slow down the rate of energy loss. You will have to do less work, which means less heat will be produced. At this point avoid as much heat loss to the environment as possible by adding clothing and/or seeking shelter.

Keep Clothing Dry

Every effort should be made to have dry clothing on. Jackets should be closed, hats and mittens donned, and hoods raised if they are available. If a member of the party is reaching exhaustion, he should be provided the clothing to prevent heat loss. If jackets are not adequate to prevent cold penetration (which means a heat loss is occurring), shelter from wind must be sought.

Replace Wet Clothing

Wet clothing must be replaced. Regardless of fabric, wet clothing will not insulate as well as dry. Use of the new synthetics will minimize heat loss if the garment is wet, but will not prevent loss of heat from the latent heat of vaporization. Remember, it will take 245 kcal (1,000 kJ) of heat to evaporate 1 pound (.45 kilograms) of water. As wet clothing can be carrying several pounds of water, the importance of preventing further heat loss due to evaporation is apparent.

Cover to Insulate Wet Clothing

If the wet clothing cannot be replaced, it must be covered with a layer of non-breathing material, such as a plastic rain suit, to prevent evaporation. It is very important to also place an insulation layer over this rain suit to prevent the increased conduction of heat through the wet fabric from further allowing a rapid heat loss.

A rain suit cover could also act as a windbreaker to help contain convection heat loss. Its use in preventing evaporation over damp clothing during a rescue operation has merit only if additional insulation is placed over the rain suit. A rain suit over insulation that is dry, however, may at times be detrimental due to the accumulation of moisture, thus decreasing the thermal efficiency of the underlying garments.

Increase Heat Production

The greatest increase of internal heat production occurs with volitional activity, that is, doing the work of walking, skiing, chopping wood, etc. If a person feels himself becoming cold, is relatively rested, has work to do or feels that he may exercise without undue loss of energy reserves, then volitional work is an excellent method of increasing the core temperature. Simply put: If you feel yourself getting chilly or starting to shiver, you may either put on more clothes, get out of the cold weather, or become active enough that you no longer feel cold.

Field Treatment of Chronic Hypothermia

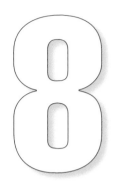

T his important subject must be divided into several topics. The first is a look at the methods that are available for adding heat to an individual under various conditions. The second is the very important distinction that must be made between mild and profound chronic hypothermia. The ideal treatment of these two conditions differs. Mild hypothermics have a core temperature that ranges between 95°F (35°C) and 90°f (32°C). Profoundly hypothermic individuals have depressed their core temperature below 90°F (32°C). They have a caloric debt of about 500 kcal. It takes about 60 kcal to rewarm a profoundly hypothermic patient by 1°F.

Heat Replacement Methods

Heat Replacement by Fluids

A liter (1.05 quarts) of intravenous solution heated to 110°F (43.3°C), which is about as warm as it can be given, would contribute 17 kcal of heat to a person with a core temperature of 90°F (32°C).

The profoundly chronic hypothermia victim is in a dehydrated state. A chronic hypothermic with a core temperature of 90°F (32°C) has a deficit of 5.5 liters (5.8 quarts) pulled mostly from the interstitial tissue, some from cell fluids, and the rest from the vascular system. The resuscitation of this individual will require replacing fluid, but the control of electrolytes, blood sugar, and acid-base balance will limit the rate of the IV Therapy. If the entire 5.5 liters of warmed fluid were infused, it would replace only a little over 90 kcal to a person who requires 500 kcal to be brought back to normal core temperature. The use of heated IV fluids in the wilderness situation is generally impractical, except with special IV heating systems that have been developed for rescue and military use.

If the victim is conscious, warm fluids may be given by mouth. But as can be guessed from the above, the amount of heat actually provided to the victim is very small. If the core temperature is 90°F (32°C), a quart of fluid heated to 140°F (65°C) will provide only 30 kcal of heat to a person who is depleted by 500 kcal. And the amount of heated fluid that the victim will be able to intake is obviously limited.

A method of providing large volumes of heated fluid, readily available in most emergency rooms, is the technique of peritoneal dialysis. Using sterile techniques, special catheters are inserted into the abdominal cavity, taking care not to penetrate the intestines or other vital organs. A liter of fluid with a starting temperature of 110.3°F (43.5°C) is then flushed through the abdominal cavity. Since the abdominal organs receive 25 percent of the cardiac output under resting condition, bathing them in warm fluid provides adequate contact with the core circulation. At a flow rate of 5 liters per hour, the patient will obtain 85 kcal/hr. Tight medical control of the content and temperature of these solutions and of the patient must be maintained during this procedure. The benefits of the technique, besides availability in most emergency rooms, is that it provides heat without fluid overload. It also is a useful means of removing many drugs that urban hypothermic victims may have taken, which is frequently a cause for their spending the night outside and becoming hypothermic in the first place.

Heat Replacement by Inhaled Air

The use of heated, humidified oxygen has been advocated to assist in the rewarming process. Heated, humidified oxygen can be tolerated as warm as 116°F (47°C), but it is generally administered at about 105°F (40°C). This technique has become one of the most important methods of adding heat to the chronic hypothermic victim in the field by rescuers in western Canada and the United States.

The amount of heat that this technique can replace is directly related to the rate and volume of breathing, the temperature of the heated mist, and to heat gain from the latent heat of vaporization as the water vapor condenses in the lungs.

To increase the amount of heat provided by heated, humidified oxygen, the patient can be intubated—that is, a tube placed into the trachea or windpipe, and the breathing rate and depth controlled by a respirator. Achieving maximum settings with this equipment would generally allow an inspired air temperature of 113°F (45°C) with a tidal volume of 20 l/min. Normal tidal volume is approximately 10 l/min, while a profoundly hypothermic victim's slower respiration rate would only result in approximately 3 l/min. If the patient had a core temperature of 82.4°F (28°C), there could be a calculated heat gain of 46 kcal/hr. If this were the only source of additional heat for the victim, even at this maximal rate, this technique would allow a temperature increase of less than 1°F (.5°C) per hour.

The true value of using heated, humidified oxygen is that the warmth is delivered to a critically important area, namely to the major blood vessels at the back of the throat, neck, and upper chest. The rather small amount of heat from this source finds its way directly to the brain stem by adjacent tissue conduction and to the heart via convection from this network of major blood vessels. A small amount of heat, but in the most critical locations!

Several lightweight units used to provide heated inhalation therapy are the Hayward and Douwens' Uvic Heat Treat System (Thermo-Genesis International, Inc.) and the Hypothermia Oxygen Warmer (Bow/Pharm, Inc.), which have made this system practical under field conditions for search and rescue teams.

An emergency approach in the field is simply to avoid further heat loss by having the victim rebreathe his own air through a wool scarf, etc. If the victim is placed with a rescuer in a sleeping bag, positioning both of their heads beneath the bag outlet salvages the respiratory heat and provides a source of heated, humidified air.

Heat Replacement by Radiation

Radiant heat is a source of heat that we often utilize, frequently without realizing it. Heat from the infrared spectrum of sunlight provides a direct source of warmth. Since they are highly reflective, snow, water, and sand increase radiant heat considerably. Even on cold days, particularly in areas sheltered from wind currents, the warmth of the sun can be a pleasant sensation.

The use of a reflecting fire, a standard technique in the old woodcraft days, and shown in Figure 8-1, was worth constructing because of the amount of heat reflected forward from the fire, providing warmth for the fireside observer as well as the cook pot or spit.

The following are all methods of adding heat via radiant energy: the formation of a hollow in the snow to protect from wind and aid in reflection of heat from the sun or external fire source; the use of metallized plastic sheeting for heat gathering and reflection; the use of infrared heat sources (such as the Coleman type radiant heater); and the use of radiant energy from heated stones and stoves. The use

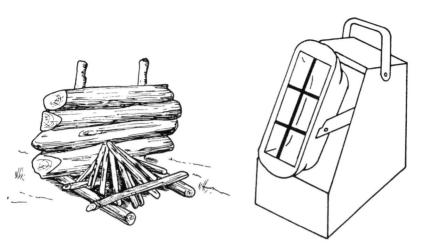

Figure 8-1

The Reflecting Fire

The traditional method of building a wood reflecting fire, this technique provides a substantial increase in the amount of heat directed forward.

of radiant heat can be helpful in select circumstances when treating hypothermia, but it should never be used for thawing frostbite victims. It must be cautiously used whenever the skin is numb from cold, for radiation heat from close sources can easily result in burns.

Heat Replacement by Conduction

Conductive heat sources must be carefully utilized or burns may result. Placing a warm rock against the victim is a conductive heat transfer, while placing it near him would be a safer, yet less intense, radiant heat transfer. Conduction can cause burns, particularly when the victim is unconscious or the skin is numb.

Immersing the victim in warm water is an example of a profound method of initiating rapid heat transfer. Indeed, this is the method of choice, when available, for the acute hypothermic victim. It may be safely used for the chronic hypothermia patient only if the rescuers are capable of maintaining tight metabolic control, as the rapid increase in body temperature will result in major alterations of blood flow, glucose, electrolyte, and other metabolic patterns. The blood levels for these items must be determined and adjusted every fifteen minutes if warm water immersion is to be "safely" used.

For the profound chronic hypothermic, it is too rapid and can result in rewarming shock due to the victim's dehydrated condition. Avoid it in the wilderness setting.

Two methods of providing heat by conduction during rescue in the field have been shown to be useful recently. One is immersion of hands and feet in warm water (113°F, 45°C), a technique advocated for some time by the Danish Navy. It takes advantage of the fact that blood travels down deep arteries in the arms and legs to the hands and feet, crosses over to the vein system through direct connections (called the deep palmar and deep plantar arches) and returns to the body by a deep vein system. Warming the hands and feet directly is a method of sending heat to the core without rewarming the outer surface of the arms or legs. In other words, this is a form of core rewarming. This seems to make intuitive sense, for when you are very cold and approach a fire, the tendency is not to open your coat to obtain heat, but to immediately face your palms towards the fire.

Another system of sending heat to the core, called *negative pressure rewarming,* is being developed: the arms are inserted into a chamber; vacuum is applied and a heating element is activated. This system promotes additional heat exchange to the core via the same physiology as above. This new device has been shown to increase the warming rate in mild hypothermia, but is not effective in profoundly hypothermic people. Watch my Web site for new information on these products (www.adventure-media.com/hypothermia/).

Heat Replacement by Convection

Warm air currents provide heat via convection. Generally, the use of warm air currents to replace heat is not a practical technique for rescue work. It supposes that air can be heated and forced past the victim. If she is damp, this method will result in an evaporative heat loss, so every precaution should be made to dry the subject thoroughly. If the air is warm enough, the consumption of energy to allow the evaporation of water from damp clothing will come from the hot air and not from the victim's diminished heat stores. Because of this, with an adequate amount of warm air, it is safe to dry and warm her simultaneously. Care must be taken not to cause burns in vulnerable, numb skin using convection reheating techniques.

Research completed during 1998 in Canada has demonstrated the ability of forced hot air to rapidly reheat a victim in the field. While two such devices have been developed, they will be practical only for use by Search and Rescue (SAR) teams due to the power requirement. The secret of their success has been the amount of heat that they deliver. It has to be high enough to make up for the fact that the warming of the skin will extinguish the shiver reflex.

Field Management of Mild Chronic Hypothermia

First, remember what constitutes a "chronic" hypothermic. It is the occurrence of hypothermia, or the lowering of the core temperature to 95°F (35°C), over a period of six hours or longer. This means that some victims of cold water immersion who, due to the temperature and their clothing, have taken longer than six hours to become hypothermic, are really chronic hypothermics with the dehydration, exhaustion, and other physiological changes characteristic of this disorder, and they are not acute (sometimes called "immersion") hypothermics. Conversely, a person falling into a glacier crevasse, hanging from a rope being drenched in melting ice water, could rapidly become hypothermic (within two hours). In such a case, that person must be considered and treated as an acute or immersion hypothermic (see page 73).

The mild chronic hypothermic has a core temperature of 95°F (35°C). This person is exhausted, but not terribly dehydrated. The victim is ataxic at this point, which means that there has been a loss of coordination to the point that such a victim will not be able to walk a 30-foot (10-meter) straight line. Mentation may be suboptimal, but this may be difficult to detect. Other signs and symptoms of mild chronic hypothermia are indicated in Table 7-1 on page 55.

The treatment required is to prevent further heat loss, provide adequate shelter or clothing, nutrition, water, rest, and heat. The form of heat and the rate of heating is not important in the mild, chronic hypothermic, but taking each of the above steps, if possible, is necessary to prevent the condition from deteriorating into profound chronic hypothermia.

If a member of your party is cold and exhausted, forcing him to walk or otherwise perform activities to heat himself from the core out will not work. The exhausted person will have too little energy substrate reserve to allow this technique to work for long. It is mandatory in these cases to take every measure possible to prevent further heat loss in this individual. The exhausted person needs protection from further heat loss; he will also need rest and nutrition so that his energy substrates can be replenished over the next several hours, and external heat, if that is convenient.

Shivering and vasoconstriction are not indicators of impending hypothermia. These activities represent the body fine-tuning its heat conservation and heat production. Uncontrolled shivering is an indicator of hypothermia, as opposed to mild shivering in response to cold air on the skin or the initial phases of mild hypothermia. If the person has limited energy stores and volitional work or shivering is not desirable, additional insulation must be acquired or other protection from the environment sought.

Field Management of Profound Chronic Hypothermia

As mentioned elsewhere, it is difficult to assess the state of hypothermia from symptoms. The symptoms of deepening hypothermia noted in Table 7-1 (page 55), include indicators of profound hypothermia. The person who has dulled reflexes, is unable to shiver, and is very clumsy is dangerously hypothermic. This person will need help in order to survive.

Helping the profound hypothermic victim to survive in the field is not an easy task. Frequently the circumstances are such that both rescuer and victim are in severe weather circumstances and both may be in danger. In helping the severely hypothermic, or the person at risk of becoming severely hypothermic, it is essential that further heat loss be prevented. Wet clothing must be handled as mentioned above.

As indicated elsewhere, the use of hot liquids (if the victim is capable of swallowing) and providing candy or other nutrients to the victim will do little immediate good, but they are critical for the long-term survival of the patient. It is extremely important to get the victim into a warm environment. The warm water given will help with the important problem of dehydration; nutrients will eventually provide a source of energy; rest will allow the by-products of energy production to be cleansed from the muscle tissues and new high-energy substrates to be formed from the nutrients that have been consumed.

Frequently the best shelter available in the field for a severely hypothermic victim will be a sleeping bag. If the victim is wet and must be transported as a litter case, remove his wet clothes and place him in a sleeping bag for transport. If his clothes cannot be removed, cover him with a waterproof cover, such as a rain suit, and place him in the sleeping bag. He will continue to cool under these circumstances if he is profoundly hypothermic.

People with a core temperature under 90°F (32°C) have generally consumed most readily available energy substrate. They are unable to produce heat from muscle shiver or work contraction. Their basal metabolic rate has been slowed and they will produce very little heat to combat the simple equilibration of cold from the extremities. They will experience an afterdrop from convection loss of heat from the core to their cold mantle and extremities and from convection loss from blood flow to their extremities. The so-called metabolic icebox in which they find themselves is a very unfriendly place. Further deterioration can be expected if gentle heat replacement does not take place.

Profound hypothermics must be handled gently to avoid agitating their very irritable hearts. The slightest jar can cause a deadly ventricular fibrillation that will effectively stop their circulation and lead to a total cardiac standstill. If CPR is initiated, it must be continued until cardiac activity is regained, which frequently means throughout the remainder of the rescue operation.

In the field with a very hypothermic victim, one who is probably below 90°F (32°C), careful rewarming as well as protection from further heat loss must be undertaken. The use of heated, aerosol mist or oxygen has been mentioned and should be used whenever available. Air rebreathing techniques, such as breathing inside of a sleeping bag, can also help minimize heat loss.

Placing carefully wrapped warm water bottles, chemical heat packs, or other warmed objects next to the neck, armpits, flanks, and groin can help stabilize heat loss. An interesting approach being studied in Scandinavia is the placement of heat packs in the palms of both hands. The rationale is that much of the blood flowing into the arms will be returning via the palmar connections of the arteries and veins. Heat in the palms might help increase the warmth of this returning blood and not induce surface vasodilation in the remainder of the arms. It also seems compatible with the natural inclination to warm one's palms by a fire when cold.

Sometimes the *cuddle technique* offers the only solution. On all expeditions into the far north, during winter or summer, I take the precaution of bringing at least one set of semi-rectangular sleeping bags that twin. The warmest bag for weight is a mummy bag, as there is minimal extra space to heat. A semi-rectangular has more weight and inside space that must be heated by the occupant. But it also provides room in which to maneuver into and out of clothes. When it's –40°, and there is no heat for the tent, dressing and undressing inside a sleeping bag prevents considerable heat loss. It also can provide a method of hypothermia rescue under remote conditions.

With the sleeping bags twinned, place the victim inside and have the rescuer crawl in to undress both the victim and himself. This process takes time and energy, allowing heat to develop. A twinned bag is large enough to allow a second rescuer to enter and similarly remove outer clothing. The second rescuer is a valuable help, as this additional thermal mass will aid the rewarming process with greater safety and less energy drain from the rescuers.

Rescuer(s) and victim should huddle together. Hat, scarf, or other clothing should be lightly wrapped around the face or used to plug the entrance of the bag to help capture warm breath and prevent the breathing of cold air. Straddling the trunk will not waste valuable heat on the extremities, which are vasoconstricted and which will slowly rewarm inside the bag anyway. Significant afterdrop should not occur due to the extremity rewarming process, but will actually be decreased from the additional heat provided by the rescuer(s). Without this outside source of heat, the hypothermic victim with a profound core temperature depression may simply continue the cooling process, lacking adequate metabolic activity.

When in doubt how hypothermic a person may be, treat as if he were profoundly hypothermic. Treat very gently, prevent further heat loss, arrange evacuation, and provide rewarming in a slow, controlled manner such as indicated above.

Managing the Cold Heart

It was noted that many victims of hypothermia were arriving in emergency rooms, profoundly cold but alive, only to die during the attempted rewarming. Postmortem examinations of hypothermic victims reveal a variety of pathological changes, but the exact cause of death has been a hotly debated subject.

The heart appears particularly vulnerable, with very slow heart rates developing as the core temperature lowers. Generally the heart rate may be expected to decrease ten beats per minute for every degree Fahrenheit of core temperature drop. An irregular heart rate called atrial fibrillation is frequent in cold hearts. By itself this arrhythmia poses no threat to life. However, as core temperature drops the heart may suddenly go into ventricular fibrillation. This arrhythmia causes the heart to fail to provide any effective pumping action. Worse, ventricular fibrillation soon degenerates into a total heart standstill or asystole—cardiac death.

While it is known that cold predisposes the heart to ventricular fibrillation, many events can initiate it. The slightest jar can produce such a lethal event, so gentle handling of all hypothermia victims is mandatory. Tickling the throat may produce ventricular fibrillation through a pharyngeal reflex. Some authorities have warned that drinking hot liquid would possibly be enough to produce it, but this seems to be more of a theoretical concern than a true problem. Certainly CPR would cause a profound chance of ventricular fibrillation and for that reason, once initiated, CPR must be continued until the victim is shown to have a functioning, regular pulse rate or acceptable electrocardiogram tracing.

The normal methods of electric countershock to start a heart will not work in hearts with a temperature below 85°F (30°C). A cold heart must be warmed to above that temperature to start it with DC countershock. If CPR has been started, it must be continued until DC countershock can be given and the heart restarted.

Currently several authorities, in conjunction with the Wilderness Medical Society, have proposed modifications of the American Heart Association's CPR standards for hypothermia. It is considered best to initiate CPR in chronic hypothermia unless:

1. Any signs of life are present.

2. Do-not-resuscitate status is documented and verified.

3. Obviously lethal injuries are present.

4. Chest wall depression is impossible.

5. Rescuers are endangered by evacuation delays or altered triage conditions. Many authorities would also add to the above criteria.

6. When beyond the roadhead, do not start CPR unless it can be continued throughout the remainder of the evacuation process.

Warnings!

Some very important "do not use as treatment" points should be made for the profoundly hypothermic victim. Never try to cool the extremities or use tourniquets. Do not use cold IVs, cold ventilation therapy, or cold treatments of any kind, including unheated oxygen. Watch what you say or do while working on patients who are unconscious or require CPR. These patients frequently remember what is done and said, which can produce severe psychological problems later on. Do not rub or manipulate the extremities. Do not give coffee or alcohol. Do not put this patient in a shower or bath.

Detection and Prevention of Acute Hypothermia

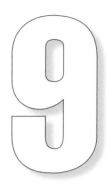

T here are several rules of thumb to predict significant risk from acute hypothermia. By definition, acute hypothermia is the result of a cooling to a core temperature of below 95°F (35°C) within two hours. Generally this will occur through cold water immersion. If the sum of the water temperature and the air temperature (in degrees Fahrenheit) is 100 or less (38 or less in degrees Celsius), there is a significant chance of developing hypothermia if a person becomes immersed.

More precisely, the risk of developing acute hypothermia can be derived from using the rate of cooling tables shown in Figure 9-1.

When unconsciousness has been reached, the person will certainly drown. Dr. Alan Steinman developed a table demonstrating the lengths of time to incapacity, unconsciousness, and cardiac arrest, under varying conditions; see Table 9-1. Note significant variations in lengths of time until loss of coordination and probable death by drowning will occur.

Various factors affect this rate of cooling. As already indicated, the temperature of the water is of significant importance. Individual body variation is very important, with cooling occurring much more rapidly for thin people than for fatter people. Children cool more quickly than adults due to their larger surface area to mass ratio. The table also indicates the importance protective clothing can have in reducing the rate of heat loss.

The use of alcohol increases the chance of acute, immersion hypothermia in several ways. Loss of coordination and improper activities or increased risk-taking are the most significant.

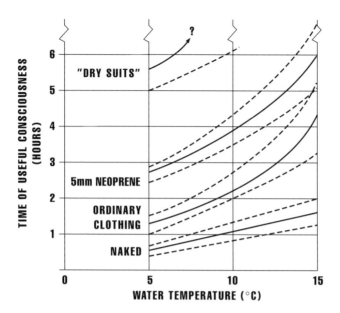

Figure 9-1

Cold Water Survival

The time of useful consciousness in hours depends on various water temperatures and conditions of dress.

The behavior of the victim in water is very important. Exercise in cold water can increase cooling rates by 35 to 50 percent. Some authorities have felt this was due to increased blood flow in muscle, while others feel it is the increased turbulence of the water that increases the rate of cooling. Regardless, movement such as swimming in water decreases survival time. Depending on circumstances, perhaps swimming to a nearby point of rescue is the best option. But for those who must remain in the water until rescue arrives, remaining as still as possible is the best choice.

Cold stress acclimatization and food intake have little effect on the rapid heat loss experienced during immersion in cold water.

Prevention of Acute Hypothermia

As mentioned, the level of activity is important. Also it is important to remove as much of your body from the cold water as possible. Even in cold wind and spray, you will lose less heat than if you remain immersed in water. Make every effort to raise yourself up out of the water on something floating; hopefully even extricate yourself onto a life raft, if possible.

Estimated Survival Times of Lean Subjects* Wearing Various Types of Protective Clothing in Rough Seas at 6.1°C.
Estimated Survival Time (hrs.)
(95% confidence range)

Clothing type	Time to Incapacity (T=34°C)	Time to Unconsciousness (T=30°C)	Time to Cardiac Arrest (T=25°C)
Control (a)	0.4–1.3	0.8–2.6	1.3–4.3
Torn, non-foam insulated dry coverall (b)	0.9–2.7	1.6–5.2	2.5–8.4
Closed-cell foam insulated, wet coverall (c)	1.0–2.9	1.9–6.0	3.0–9.9
Closed-cell foam insulated, custom fitted wet-suit (d)	1.6–4.7	3.1–9.9	4.9–16.2
Intact, non-foam insulated dry coverall (e)	2.9–8.8	5.7–18.2	9.1–30.0

* Body fat = 11.1%
(a) Lightweight clothing
(b) Identical to (e) with 2" tear in left shoulder
(c) 3.2 mm thick insulation in loose-fitting coverall
(d) 4.8 mm thick insulation; tight fitting
(e) Watertight shell over thick, fiberfill, insulated underwear

Table 9-1

Estimated Survival Time

(From Steinman, *Wilderness Medicine Newsletter*, Vol. 7, No 2, April 1990.)

Several years ago a new technique to allow long-term survival in the water was developed called *drownproofing*. This was a technique of flotation that minimized the movements made, thus conserving energy. It is a breath-holding maneuver, using minimal kicking strokes to return the victim to the surface to raise her face to air and grab a quick breath. The action of blowing out air and raising the head normally causes the person to sink under water. As she has fully expanded lungs, she will soon float to the surface—where the process is repeated. Drownproofing is a valuable personal skill that I have been able to teach to many of my Boy Scouts without difficulty.

Unfortunately the frequent submersion of the head required in using the drownproofing technique increases heat loss in cold water. It has been estimated that a person using drownproofing in 50°F (10°C) water will have an average survival time of one and one-half hours. Treading and swimming in the same temperature water might extend survival to a little over two hours. Holding still in a personal flotation device (life jacket) could increase the survival time to almost three hours. A technique of assuming a curled up position in a life jacket, called HELP (Heat Escape Lessening Posture), may extend survival time in the same temperature water to over four hours.

A similar heat-preserving technique has been designed for two or more people with life jackets in the water—the HUDDLE position. By placing the life jackets on backwards, people can hug each other so that the chest, groin, and legs can be pressed together, thus preserving some of the body heat from the cold convection currents.

While the HELP and HUDDLE techniques seem theoretically beneficial, controlled experiments at the University of Minnesota Medical School at Duluth have failed to demonstrate the expected difference in core cooling rate of either. Dr. Pozos, a respected authority in hypothermia research, feels this is due to the technical difficulty of performing these maneuvers. He advises practicing the HELP position with the same life jacket that you might be using in the cold water. With many models and varying body builds, the person assuming the curled up position will roll in the water, allowing repeated cold water exposure to the head and back of the neck. This causes more of a heat loss through this area than one saves from decreasing the abdominal/groin heat loss. If in assuming the HELP position you find yourself rolling around or awash with cold water, Dr. Pozos recommends simply crossing your legs at the ankles and bringing the thighs together. This should minimize heat loss, while not allowing you to go awash in the water.

The HUDDLE position can be very difficult to achieve since each member needs to be balanced with regard to his or her flotation level and size. People tend to float at different levels, even with life jackets on. An unbalanced group constantly allows members to go awash and requires excessive struggling to keep in balance. Prior dunking practice with the same HUDDLE group is again impossible to achieve normally, but almost essential for this technique to work adequately. The best aspect of the HUDDLE method is that it keeps a group together for psychological benefit and may aid a rescue. If a HUDDLE group finds itself going awash, rearrange the group or break up into smaller groups.

A technique that has saved the lives of many people who have found themselves trapped aboard a sinking ship in cold waters has been for them to put on as many layers of clothing as they could find. If possible, the outerlayer should be covered with a rain suit to decrease the effects of conduction currents. A large life jacket then covers the rain suit. These simple measures can extend your cold water survival time considerably.

Field Treatment of Acute Hypothermia and Submersion

10

F alling into cold water will rapidly induce hypothermia. This "acute" or "immersion" hypothermia has many characteristics that are different from the slowly developing "chronic" hypothermia of cold weather exposure. Survival is dependent on the water and air temperature, protective clothing, body size and percentage of body fat of the victim, activity, evidence of near drowning, and resources of the rescuers.

There are three primary ways in which death can occur during cold water immersion. As cold water will conduct heat at a rate of twenty to twenty-five times that of air at the same temperature, the most common problem will be a continual cooling, resulting in possible confusion at a core temperature of about 95°F (35°C) and unconsciousness at roughly 90°F (32°C), with subsequent drowning. Others may abruptly drown from a reflexive involuntary gasping of the icy water. More rarely, the sudden shock of ice water entry may cause immediate cardiac death from ventricular fibrillation.

When rescuing an immersion hypothermic victim, it is very important to prevent any rough handling, as the heart will be very sensitive and ventricular fibrillation may be accidentally induced. This is true of the victim who is walking, talking, and in every way behaving normally. After prolonged cold water immersion, this victim must be made to lie down and treated as a litter case. Vasoconstriction

Hypothermia **73**

will have allowed his or her skin temperature to cool as low as the water temperature, while the core temperature may be quite high, even above 95°F (35°C). Equilibration of this temperature will result in a profound core cooling.

Core cooling during immersion, and afterdrop of the core temperature after removal from cold water, occurs by two mechanisms: conduction loss of heat through adjacent cold tissues and convection cooling by blood flow through cold tissues. The relative contribution of these two modes of cooling depends upon the anatomical portion of the core under consideration. The pelvic region probably cools primarily through conduction heat loss into the thigh and gluteal muscles, with a smaller convection loss due to blood flow from the legs. It is also well known that stool in the rectum can remain cold and cause considerable errors when comparing rectal temperatures with core temperatures near the heart. The heart area in the middle of the chest probably cools less from the conduction loss of heat through the lungs than it does from cold blood return from the extremities, to include the head and neck.

If the victim is actively moving around, the convection loss from blood flow to the extremities will cause a considerable afterdrop, which may well precipitate a lethal cardiac arrhythmia.

The controversy in the care of the profound, acute hypothermic is the use of hot water (110°F or 43°C) immersion. The profound heat deficit from which these people are suffering has led many rescuers to employ this rapid reheating method. The rapid reheating would induce increased blood flow to the extremities, but it also adds heat to the neck, flanks, and femoral areas to help warm cooler returning blood, as well as provide massive amounts of heat to the entire skin surface. If the victim is suffering from dehydration, which may well be the case after an immersion period of two hours or longer, the potential of vascular collapse absolutely contraindicates using this technique.

Hot water immersion is the technique employed primarily in Denmark where they have had extensive experience with acute immersion hypothermia from North Sea disasters during wartime and most recently from oil drilling platform accidents.

The Danish experience has been that people do better with the hot water immersion technique. It is likely that the very cold extremities of slowly reheated people will cause more of an afterdrop via both convection and conduction equilibration than seen with the rapid reheating technique. Hot water immersion may rapidly rewarm the entire mantle layer and lead to less of an afterdrop during the heat equilibration process.

In the field, tubs of hot water will probably not be available unless a cabin or other facility is nearby. Constructing a bonfire provides an alternate source of massive heat. Lacking the ability to start a large rewarming fire, the use of cuddling may be the only alternative. The survivor should be partially disrobed and placed in a sleeping bag with one, or preferably two, lightly clad rescuers. The victim may not feel the necessity of such careful treatment, but attentive rewarming with an outside heat source is best. If only a mummy style sleeping bag is available, dry the victim and place him in the bag. He may be given warm liquids by mouth, but expect a core temperature afterdrop due to the tremendous amount of cold in the mantle, which must equilibrate with the warmer core. Clothes may be warmed and placed in the bag with the victim. Care should be taken with objects that might contact the person and cause thermal burns on the numb and delicate skin. Bottles of warm water, chemical heat packs, and warmed objects should be carefully padded.

If the person has experienced cold water immersion when the air temperature is subzero, it will frequently be impossible to remove the frozen clothes. When alone, the victim may roll in the snow, which will freeze to the outer clothing and form an icy shell to provide some wind and thermal protection. This is a desperate situation and finding a warm shelter or building a fire may be the only chance for survival. On several occasions I have had members of my party, myself included, fall through ice in freezing temperatures. We never rolled in the snow, but each time our clothes rapidly froze. Fortunately we were able to get a massive fire started to totally warm and dry ourselves. Once, two members of my expedition beat a hasty retreat in their frozen clothes to the cabin they had just left. They were able to make a fire in the stove rapidly, as they had prepared the wood prior to their departure. After prolonged immersion, this rapid movement can be lethal, as was mentioned in the case of the Danish fishermen (page 9). But when there are no other choices, warmth must be earnestly sought before the numbing effect of the cold makes action impossible. Cold water immersion in subfreezing, and certainly in subzero, temperatures is a desperate situation. What people do not recognize is the danger cold water immersion has even when the air temperature is above freezing.

Cliff Jacobson in his book *Canoeing Wild Rivers* (ICS Books, 1989) relates a tragic death of a famous and highly experienced expedition canoeist in 1955 on the Dubawnt river in the Northwest Territories: In his story "Death on the Barrens" (John Long, ed., *Close Shaves*, The Globe Pequot Press, 1997) George Grinnell describes the desperate circumstances surrounding his party's accident in raging cold water rapids, resulting in the death of the expedition leader, Arthur Moffat in

1955. The crew, which lost virtually all of its equipment, barely survived the mass wetting: Moffat was comatose and another crew member, Joe, was severely hypothermic. One of the crew crawled into a sleeping bag with Joe. There was no one who could crawl into a bag with Arthur. Joe survived; Arthur did not. Arthur was so hypothermic from this dunking that it is possible he might not have survived, but this cuddling was perhaps the only chance that he had. By the time it was tried later, they were convinced that he was dead.

The death of Moffat is even more ironic if one is aware of another event that also took place in the barrens of the far north, but over 130 years before.

An early recorded testimony to the value of cuddling a hypothermic victim dates back to an early journal of Arctic exploration. Dr. Richardson, a physician on the Sir John Franklin Expedition to the Hood River in Arctic Canada in 1821, directed the rescue of a party member who had capsized in an icy rapids. The account reads: "Belanger was suffering extremely, immersed to his middle in the center of the rapid, the temperature of which was very little above the freezing point, the upper part of his body covered with wet clothes, exposed in a temperature not much above zero, to a strong breeze.... By direction of Dr. Richardson, he was instantly stripped, and being rolled up in blankets, two men undressed themselves and went to bed with him; but it was some hours before he recovered his warmth and sensations." *Narrative of a Journey to the Shores of the Polar Sea in the Years 1819, 20, 21* by Sir John Franklin (1823). Cuddling is a poor way to transfer heat, as both persons are cylinders with the heat transfer occurring only on a thin segment of each body. If one or both are hypothermic, the vasoconstriction produces the effect of forming an insulation layer between the warmer core temperatures and cold skin layer. The heat transfer between rescuer and victim is improved by having both individuals breathe only inside the bag, thus exchanging heat by respiration (see page 59).

Cold Water Submersion

Cold water submersion is always associated with asphyxiation and simultaneous hypothermia. The asphyxiation results in brain death so the prompt rescue and immediate implementation of CPR play an important role in the survival of the victim. Total submersion in cold water causes rapid core cooling, which results in lower oxygen demand by the brain and other body tissues and increases the change of survival over that of a victim of warm water submersion. These rapid cooling rates in very cold water submersion are due to the normal conduction and convection losses of heat as experienced by the cold water immersion victim, increased losses from the submerged head with its large unprotected blood flow, and, to a less extent, from core cooling due to cold water swallowing and pulmonary aspiration.

Children are cooled more rapidly than adults due to their large surface area to mass ratio. They frequently have less subcutaneous fat for insulation than an adult. And in children up to the age of two or three, there at times can exist a circulatory reflex called the "mammalian diving reflex." The immersion of the child's face triggers this reflex, which causes oxygenated blood to move from the lungs to the heart and brain, the heart rate to slow to several beats per minute, and a shutting of the epiglottis, which protects the lungs from water while submerged. Rapid cooling decreases the tissue oxygen requirement and the brain is especially protected by the oxygen-rich blood that has been shunted to it during the initial phase of the reflex. This reflex can extend the underwater survival for children to slightly beyond thirty minutes.

Older persons resuscitated successfully are probably not beneficiaries of the mammalian diving reflex, but of the rapidly induced hypothermia of cold water submersion. Full recovery after ten to forty minutes of submersion can occur, even in adults. Because of this, CPR must be immediately started in all apparently drowned immersion and submersion hypothermia victims and continued aggressively.

Do not warm the submersion victim during field treatment, which consists solely of CPR, but do not cool the victim further, either. Provide a thermal wrap that will prevent further heat loss to the environment. Continue CPR until paramedical or EMT personnel assume responsibility for the victim or until exhaustion overtakes the rescuers.

Victims should be transferred to hospitals with specialized experience with this problem, but the victim will never have a chance if rescuers do not implement CPR immediately.

Frostbite and Other Cold-Related Injuries

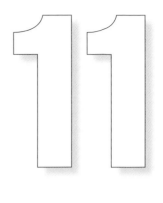

Frostbite is the freezing of tissue. Surface skin goes through several phases before this occurs. The freezing process requires predisposing risk factors to be present before the events leading to frostbite are initiated.

Outside temperatures must be below freezing for frostbite to occur. The underlying physical condition of the victim, length of cold contact, and type of cold contact are other important factors leading to frostbite. Skin temperature must be cooled to between 22°F and 24°F (-5.5°C and -4.4°C) before tissue will freeze.

A decreased peripheral circulation from vasoconstriction due to hypothermia can be an important factor in frostbite information, but generally even severe vasoconstriction will not be enough unless one of several other situations is present.

One is the wearing of constricting garments, such as boots that are too tight, or elastic wrist or ankle bands that are too snug. Bootliners constructed of foam material with air cells that can expand at high altitude have caused many frostbitten feet in mountaineers. Cold weather clothing should be constructed to avoid constricting bands on ankles and wrists especially.

Dehydration is a risk factor for frostbite. As indicated elsewhere, dehydration is also a risk factor for hypothermia. Dehydration will generally exist in a person suffering from chronic hypothermia.

Adequate nutrition and prevention of fatigue are additional preventative measures in the fight against frostbite. This is in large measure due to their importance in preventing hypothermia.

It is rare for a healthy person, even with reduced activity in bitter cold weather such as prolonged standing, to develop frostbite. But injury of any sort seems to allow frostbite to more easily develop. If shock is present, the risk of frostbite injury increases dramatically.

Contact with metal objects that rapidly conduct heat from the body may cause frostbite. Even a thin glove which, while allowing dexterity and not providing much insulation, would be valuable in preventing direct contact with metal hardware used in climbing, working, or camping under below freezing situations. Extreme caution with liquid fuels must be maintained as these liquids will cool to the recent average ambient temperature and will cause immediate tissue freezing in subzero conditions.

The use of substances that cause vasoconstriction, primarily smoking, should be avoided. In healthy people smoking does not appear to cause increased risk of frostbite as long as they are not smoking during the time of cold exposure. Persons sensitive to the effects of nicotine, such as those suffering from *Raynard's* or *Buerger's* disease, must absolutely quit smoking and are at risk of frostbite during freezing conditions.

Lack of adequate oxygen supply is also a factor. This is much more prevalent in high altitude climbing. It is particularly noticeable that climbing above 24, 500 feet (7,500 meters) without oxygen frequently results in extensive frostbite among even highly experienced climbing parties.

Of all the factors mentioned, hypothermia itself is the most important predisposing factor to the formation of frostbite. But a person with hypothermia may well not have frostbite, and vice versa, a person with frostbite may not be hypothermic.

Generally when frostbite occurs, it will be to feet, hands, ears, or nose. Only rarely will it occur elsewhere and then only with some unusual cause, such as metal contact, injury, etc.

As mentioned elsewhere, an important method of body heat control is the vasoconstriction of arteries to prevent warm blood flow to the surface and thus decrease heat loss. In the skin, the heat and oxygen transfer occurs in the capillary system, the microscopic vessels that connect the veins and arteries together. These thin vessels are so small that red blood cells must travel through them in single file. When the small peripheral arteries, called arterioles, clamp down, the blood flow to the capillaries ceases. Blood is shunted from the arterioles directly to small veins, venules. Oxygen and heat is no longer removed. The "*hunting reflex*," or *periodic vasodilation*, can allow periodic surges of warm blood through the capillaries to provide oxygen and heat to help prevent tissue anoxia (lack of oxygen) and freezing. But if the body core temperature drops, this episodic warming will decrease to the point that local tissue freezing may result.

If the outside temperature is below freezing, and the circulation of warm blood has been compromised, the fluid between the cells may start to freeze. This freezing process pulls additional fluid from the surrounding cells as the icy crystals grow. While these crystals do not seem to cause tissue damage, the dehydration process results in damage to the cell's internal metabolic systems and structures. This damage can become severe within half an hour.

In the case of rapid freezing, say from contact with metal or liquid fuels during bitter cold temperatures, ice crystal formation can occur both between cells and within the cells, thus more rapidly destroying these cells and preventing any chance of recovery of this injured tissue.

Traditionally several degrees of frostbite are recognized, but the initial treatment for all is the same. The actual degree of severity will not be known for an extended period of time.

By definition *frostbite* means that tissue is not only frozen, but damaged. For practical purposes, two types of frostbite are generally recognized, although some authorities say four types. The first type is *superficial frostbite*. The surface layer of skin is frozen, but deeper tissues are not. When pressing on a superficial frostbite it will be noted that while the surface is frozen and white, it will give under firm, gentle pressure as lower tissues are still pliable. In the second type, *deep frostbite*, even the deeper tissues are frozen solid. This tissue feels hard as a rock. There will be a reasonable chance for full recovery of tissue with superficial frostbite, while deep frostbite can result in considerable tissue destruction.

Once thawing has taken place, it will be impossible to use the above criteria for distinguishing superficial from deep frostbite. After thawing, the formation of blisters may be a guide to the severity of the freeze damage and can act as a prognosis to the eventual damage that may result. Blisters that form within 24 to 36 hours and are located further up the hand or leg generally indicate severe peripheral damage, and the tissue beyond that point may be dead with eventual total loss.

It is apparent that most tissue damage occurs during the reheating, or thawing, phase of frostbite. Studies of frostbite blisters show the presence of toxic radicals, thromboxane, and various prostaglandins. These substances increase the constriction of blood vessels, start blood clotting, and may directly damage cell walls. Experimental evidence suggests that starting an anti-inflammatory medication, such as aspirin, before rewarming is started might minimize this rewarming damage. Rewarming should not be delayed until an anti-inflammatory can be started, however, because the longer the limb remains frozen, the greater the resulting damage.

The specific therapy for a deep frozen extremity is rapid thawing in warm water of approximately 110°F (43°C). Take precautions to never let this water temperature be higher than 115°F (46°C) or the results will be disastrous. The thawing may take 20 to 30 minutes. It should be continued until all paleness of the tips of the toes or fingers has turned pink or burgundy red, but not longer. This will be very painful and will require pain medication at the start of the procedure. Frostbite victims should be treated for shock routinely with elevation of the feet and lowering of the head, as shock can easily occur when the frostbite victim enters a warm environment.

Frostbite injuries should be rewarmed as soon as possible upon their discovery, even if a rapid rewarming process is not available. The longer the part remains frozen, the greater the damage that will result. Many frostbite injuries thaw by themselves right in the field. Increased activity may allow a frozen foot to rewarm, with the victim incidentally discovering the purple discoloration of the thawed tissue when examining a numb foot.

Avoid opening the blisters that form unless further activity will obviously cause them to rupture. Use sterile techniques to aspirate the fluid and cover with a sterile aloe vera cream. Do not cut the skin away unless it starts to decay, but allow the blisters to eventually resolve on their own. These blisters may last two to three weeks. They must be treated with care to prevent infections (best done in a hospital by gloved attendants). The worse complication that can develop at this stage is an infection of these tissues, resulting in a "wet gangrene." Infection can cause considerable tissue loss, far beyond the area of initial freeze injury. It is important that the patient's tetanus immunization be current, certainly with the previous ten years.

A black carapace will form in severe frostbite. This is actually a form of dry gangrene. This carapace will gradually fall off with amazingly good results beneath. Efforts to hasten carapace removal generally result in infection, delay in healing, and increased loss of tissue. Leave these blackened areas alone. The black carapace separation can take over six months, but it is worth the wait. Without surgical intervention most frostbite wounds heal in six months to a year. At times, emergency surgery is indicated in freeze injuries. After thawing, tissue swelling can become so profound that the remaining circulation may be compromised. Surgery to relieve this pressure, called a fasciotomy, must be performed. The necessity for this procedure is indicated by sophisticated methods of blood flow and tissue pressure analysis.

If a frozen member has been thawed and the patient must be transported, use cotton between toes (or fluff sterile gauze and place between the toes) and cover other areas with a loose sterile bandage to protect the skin during sleeping bag/stretcher evacuation. If a fracture also exists, immobilize when in the field, loosely so as not to impair the circulation any further. Carefully avoid refreezing, which will cause substantial additional tissue loss.

Frost Nip

Frost nip, or superficial surface freezing, can be readily treated in the field, if recognized early enough. By watching for and immediately responding to frost nip, permanent damage to tissue can be avoided.

Frost nip is most common on the ears and the tip of the nose. When frost nip is suspected, thaw immediately so that it does not become more serious frostbite. Warm the hands by blowing on them, placing them as fists within mittens, or withdrawing them into the parka through the sleeves. Avoid opening the front of the parka to minimize heat loss.

It is difficult to evaluate the existence of frost nip on feet. A good clue is the loss of sensation in the toes and foot, which should mandate examination if sensation cannot be readily restored by increasing activity or stomping of the feet. Feet should be thawed against a companion or cupped in your own hands in a roomy sleeping bag, or otherwise placed in contact with warm human flesh in an insulated environment.

Your own nose can be thawed by cupping your hands over your face and exhaling. Ears can be warmed by pressing warm hands over them. Your hands may have to be warmed first by blowing on them or insulting them adequately in large mittens, etc.

Frost nip can be painless and its presence should be watched for on your companions. On one of my winter trips into subarctic Canada, a 17-year-old companion almost constantly frost nipped his nose whenever the temperature fell below -20°F (-29°C). He was healthy, in excellent physical shape (probably the best condition of us all), and he wore arctic clothing that was identical to the rest of ours. We repeatedly had to warm him to thaw his nose, as he seemed oblivious to the fact that the tip of his nose was literally frosted white.

Cold-Induced Bronchospasm

Cold-induced bronchospasm, a form of asthma, sometimes called *frozen lung* or pulmonary chilling, occurs when breathing rapidly at very low temperatures, generally colder than -20°F (-29°C). There is burning pain, sometimes coughing of blood, and frequently asthmatic wheezing. If irritation of the diaphragm occurs, a pain in the shoulder(s) and upper stomach may develop that can last for one to two weeks.

The cause of this condition is a severe bronchial irritation. This results in bronchospasms, the formation of mucus, and possibly pulmonary infiltration resulting in the pleuritic pain.

The treatment is bed rest, steam inhalations, drinking extra water, humidification of the air being breathed, and absolutely no smoking. This problem may be avoided by using parka hoods, face masks, or breathing through mufflers that allow the rebreathing of warm, humidified air.

Immersion Foot

Immersion foot, also called trench foot, results during wet, cold conditions with temperature exposures from 68°F (20°C) down to freezing, if proper foot care is not maintained. It results from vasoconstriction of the arterioles with subsequent loss of heat and oxygen supply to surface tissues. Under prolonged exposure to wet, cold conditions, this can result in damage to the skin. The temperature need not drop below 50°F (10°C) for substantial injury to occur.

To prevent this problem avoid non-breathing (rubber) footwear when possible. Dry feet and change socks every evening. Periodically elevate, air, dry, and massage the feet to promote circulation. Avoid tight, constricting footwear or lower leg garments.

One might question the possible development of immersion foot when using a vapor barrier sock. I do not know if this has ever occurred, but it is a possibility. My companions and I have never found our liner socks to be very damp, but a mountaineering friend of mine reports wringing considerable water from his liner socks when using a vapor barrier system. In that instance, the main protection from immersion foot injury would be the maintenance of a very warm foot, made possible from a superior or protected insulation. The U.S. Army "mickey mouse" or "bunny" boots used under arctic conditions allow considerable moisture buildup. These boots are generally very warm, thus precluding the formation of immersion foot. But a precaution everyone should take when using an occlusive boot or liner system is to dry feet nightly and sooner if they feel cold.

There are two stages of immersion foot, clinically. In the first stage the foot is cold, swollen, waxy, mottled with dark burgundy to blue splotches. The foot is resilient to palpation, whereas the frozen foot is very hard. Skin is sodden and friable. Loss of feeling makes walking difficult.

Hypothermia   **83**

The second stage lasts for days to weeks. The feet become swollen, red, and hot. Blisters form, and infection and gangrene are frequently problems during this stage.

Treatment differs from frostbite and hypothermia in the following ways: (1) Give the patient 10 grains of aspirin every six hours to help decrease platelet adhesion and clotting ability of the blood; (2) Give additional stronger pain medication if necessary, but discontinue as soon as possible; (3) Provide an ounce of hard liquor (30 ml) every hour while awake and two ounces (60 ml) every two hours during sleeping hours to vasodilate and increase the blood flow to the feet.

If you are unsure whether or not you are dealing with immersion foot or frostbite, or if you may have suffered both, treat as for frostbite. The injury of immersion foot should be treated by a physician. The chance of damaging the tissue, or of serious infection, and of long-term pain and other complications is very high.

Chilblain

Chilblain, also commonly called *pernio*, and less frequently *kibe* and *chimetlon,* results from exposure of dry skin to temperatures from 60°F (15.5°C) to freezing. The skin becomes red, swollen, frequently tender, and itching. This is the least severe form of cold injury. No tissue loss ever results. Strictly speaking, the term "kibe" refers to a crack in the skin caused by cold or an ulcerated chilblain.

The cause is probably histamine release in cold traumatized tissue, resulting in further tissue irritation.

Treatment is the prevention of further exposure with protective clothing over bare skin and the use of ointments such as A & D Ointment or white petroleum jelly.

Glossary

Acute hypothermia Hypothermia of quick onset, generally six hours or less. Some authorities feel that two hours or less should be classified as "acute," while the period two to six hours should be called "prolonged or "sub-acute" hypothermia.

Afterdrop The further lowering of the core temperature after the reheating process has begun.

Ambient temperature The temperature of the environment—the so-called "outside temperature."

Arrhythmia Irregular rhythm, such as heart rate.

Asystole A heart that has stopped beating.

Ataxia Loss of coordination.

Basal metabolic rate The amount of energy required by the resting body to maintain normal physiologic functions.

Calorie The amount of heat necessary to raise 1 gram of water 1°C at 15°C.

Cerebellum The portion of the brain that controls balance and coordination, among other reflexes.

Chilblain An irritated reaction of dry skin to below freezing, damp conditions.

Chimetlon Another term for Chilblain.

Circadian The same as diurnal, changing on a 24 hour cycle.

Clo A measurement of clothing insulation.

Cold Diureses An increase in urination when exposed to cold.

Conduction The direct transfer of heat from one object to another.

Convection The transfer of heat by the movement of liquid or gas.

Core The vital interior of the body consisting of the organs, most notably the heart, lungs, and brain.

Countercurrent heat exchange A method of heat preservation whereby returning venous blood is directed to a deeper set of veins that run alongside arteries. Heat from the artery helps increase the temperature of the returning blood, while the arterial blood cools on its outward journey.

CPR Cardiopulmonary resuscitation.

Crystallizaton, latent heat of See "Fusion, latent heat of."

Diurnal Changing daily. Many body functions have a diurnal change. The resting temperature is one of them.

Drowning Death by suffocation underwater.

Drownproofing A technique of remaining afloat without a life jacket.

Endogenous Controlled or originating from within.

Equivalent chill temperature An expression in degrees of temperature that represents the feeling of cold due to the effect of wind currents.

Evaporation Changing from a liquid to a gas.

Evaporation, latent heat of The amount of heat required to change a liquid to a gas without an increase in the temperature of the substance. To evaporate water it requires 540 kcal (2,262 kJ) per kilogram (2.2 pounds).

Fibrillation Quivering. In heart muscle an arrhythmia that produces a very erratic heart rate, if it is atrial; or a potentially lethal heart arrhythmia that allows no effective blood movement, if it is ventricular.

Frost nip Superficial surface freezing of tissue.

Frostbite The freezing of tissue.

Frozen lung Not a freezing process of the lung, but a pulmonary irritation caused by very cold air.

Fusion, latent heat of The amount of heat required to melt a solid to a liquid state, such as snow to water, without raising the temperature of the substance. This equals 79.7 kcal (334 kJ) per kilogram (2.2 pounds) of ice.

HELP Heat Escape Lessening Posture, a method of heat preservation when immersed in cold water.

Homeotherm An organism, such as a mammal, that must maintain its internal body temperature within a narrow range. For humans this is 96° to 101°F (35.5° to 38°C).

HUDDLE A method of heat preservation when immersed with a group in cold water.

Hunting response A popular term for "cold-induced vasodilator," the sporadic opening of constricted blood vessels.

Hypothalamus A portion of the brain that controls temperature regulation, among other regulatory functions.

Hypothermia The lowering of the body temperature to 95°F (35°C) or lower.

Immersion In water up to the head.

Immersion foot Trench foot; a wet cold injury of the foot.

Immersion hypothermia Hypothermia from immersion in cold water. As it is very quick in onset, it is a form of acute hypothermia.

Inuit The proper name for "Eskimo" and used throughout this text. The Inuit consider the term "Eskimo" derogatory.

Joule Work done in one second by a current of one ampere against a resistance of one ohm.

Kilocalorie Sometimes called a "large calorie." A unit of metabolic measurement, the so-called "calorie" referred to in diets.

Kibe A form of chilblain with cracking of the skin.

Kcal Kilocalorie

KJ Kilojoule

Mammalian diving reflex A method of heat and oxygen conservation found in many diving mammals and some youngsters.

Mantle The outer surface layers of the body, as opposed to the body "core." The outer mantle consists of skin and subcutaneous fat. The inner mantle consists of muscle.

Metabolic icebox A term for describing the relatively stable condition of the profoundly hypothermic individual.

Microenvironment The area immediately surrounding an object.

Near drowning Survival for at least twenty-four hours after a drowning episode.

Pernio Another term for "chilblain."

Poikilotherm An animal that varies its temperature according to the surrounding temperature, the so-called cold-blooded animals and plants.

Radiation Heat transfer by the emission of infrared energy.

Specific dynamic action of food The energy used in the metabolic processing and digestion of food.

Submersion In water over the head.

Submersion hypothermia Hypothermia from submersion in cold water. As it is very quick in onset, it is a form of acute hypothermia. As the victim is underwater, it will result in near drowning or drowning.

Thermogenesis The formation of heat.

Thermoregulaton The control of temperature.

Trench foot See "immersion foot."

Vapor barrier A technique of preventing the skin from breathing and transmitting moisture to clothing or the outside atmosphere.

Vaporization, latent heat of The same as "latent heat of evaporation."

Vasoconstriction The clamping down or narrowing of blood vessels.

Vasodilatation An alternate spelling of "vasodilator."

Vasodilator The opening of blood vessels to maximum diameter.

Volitional work Work performed by desire to accomplish a task. Purposeful exercise.

Windchill factor The amount of heat lost due to convection by wind currents at specific ambient temperatures.

Index